Recreational Therapy Assessment

Thomas K. Skalko, PhD, LRT/CTRS, FDRT

East Carolina University

Jerome F. Singleton, PhD, CTRS

Dalhousie University

Editors

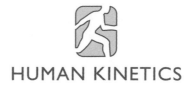

HUMAN KINETICS

Library of Congress Cataloging-in-Publication information is available. LCCN 2019019009

ISBN: 978-1-4925-5825-5 (print)

The web addresses cited in this text were current as of May 2019, unless otherwise noted.

Acquisitions Editor: Diana Vincer
Senior Developmental Editor: Melissa Feld
Managing Editor: Derek Campbell
Copyeditor: Heather Gauen Hutches
Indexer: Nancy Ball
Permissions Manager: Dalene Reeder
Graphic Designer: Denise Lowry
Cover Designer: Keri Evans
Cover Design Associate: Susan Rothermel Allen
Photographs (interior): © Rick Green, unless otherwise noted
Photo Production Manager: Jason Allen
Senior Art Manager: Kelly Hendren
Illustrations: © Human Kinetics, unless otherwise noted
Printer: Sheridan Books

Printed in the United States of America   10 9 8 7 6 5 4 3 2 1

The paper in this book is certified under a sustainable forestry program.

Human Kinetics
P.O. Box 5076
Champaign, IL 61825-5076
Website: www.HumanKinetics.com

In the United States, email info@hkusa.com or call 800-747-4457.
In Canada, email info@hkcanada.com.
In the United Kingdom/Europe, email hk@hkeurope.com.

For information about Human Kinetics' coverage in other areas of the world, please visit our website:
www.HumanKinetics.com

Tell us what you think!
Human Kinetics would love to hear what we
can do to improve the customer experience.
Use this QR code to take our brief survey.

E7182

This text is dedicated to our parents, Henry Charles and Rosemary Singleton and Andrew and Anna Skalko. Our parents supported us during our careers and supported us in the pursuit of all our passions.

To our spouses, who have put up with us during the writing of this text, Sandy Singleton and Diane Skalko.

To the children of Jerry and Sandy Singleton, Mike and Anna Singleton. and to Thom's children, Monica, Thomas Joshua, Andrew, Garrett, Sydney, and Leah. Thank you for always hanging in there across time and for providing us with laughter and enjoyment.

To our siblings who have passed way before their time, Joseph Singleton and Andrew Charles Skalko and Ann Marie Skalko, whose spirits were always present with us during our careers.

CONTENTS

We wish to acknowledge the development of the text's proposal from Ms. Andrea King, MA, CTRS, whose master's thesis assisted in identifying how CTRS practitioners framed how they perceive the assessment process, and Dr. Tristan Hopper, CTRS, who was a master's student at the time of the text's proposal and provided a student's perspective on gaps within assessment during his education.

We also feel it important to acknowledge all the authors in the text, whose insights will build capacity for TR professionals related to the assessment process for students and current TR professionals.

This text would not be possible without the support and guidance of the mentors who assisted us in our careers:

- Dr. Gerald O'Morrow, who introduced us to the APIE process and how to be therapists
- Dr. Fred Humphrey, who challenged us to think critically
- Dr. Elliot Avedon, who provided us with many of our foundations for understanding direct service delivery

- Dr. Gene Hayes, who continues to strum our softer chords in how we approach the practice and our relationships
- Dr. Stuart Schleien, our colleague for too many years to count, who helped challenge us in our thinking within the profession
- Dr. Ira Goldenberg, who taught Thom to speak freely and to engage in thoughtful, educated discussion on the who, what, and how of managing people and seeking your best

Finally, to all the Recreational Therapy students, both undergraduate and graduate, who have helped us define our mission and who have embraced the concept of challenging the status quo and reaching for your best. To all our colleagues we have worked with and all the RT practitioners we had the opportunity to interact with during our careers. Ultimately, this text is for all our colleagues, past, present, and future, who make a difference in the lives of persons with differing levels of abilities across the life course.

Framing the Text for the Reader

Thomas K. Skalko, PhD, LRT/CTRS, FDRT

Jerome F. Singleton, PhD, CTRS

Therapeutic recreation (TR) as a profession uses the Assess, Plan, Implement, and Evaluate (APIE) process to demonstrate the efficacy of recreational therapy (RT) practice. The TR educational requirements for entry to RT practice are framed within the National Council for Therapeutic Recreation Certification (NCTRC) and the Commission on Accreditation for Allied Health Education Programs' Committee on Accreditation of Recreational Therapy Education knowledge domains. The TR profession has framed service delivery within a variety of models (Austin, 1991; O'Morrow & Reynolds, 1989; Peterson & Stumbo, 2009). The assessment process frames what to plan, how to implement, and how to evaluate the services of the recreational therapist. King (2014) conducted a study of Certified Therapeutic Recreation Specialists (CTRS) and found that the process of assessment was complex (see chapter 1). King's findings provided the connection to the World Health Organization's (WHO, 2001) *International Classification of Functioning, Disabil-*

ity and Health (ICF) to assist in the classification of functioning in the assessment process.

This textbook aims to guide the therapeutic recreation profession in assessing the consumer within the context of the World Health Organization's *International Classification of Functioning, Disability and Health* (ICF). The ICF offers rehabilitation professionals, social service providers, and policy makers a means to classify the functioning of the individual in the exercise of daily living. By integrating the process of assessment with the ICF, the recreational therapy professional will be able to better focus the outcomes of their services, as well as better integrate their services with those of other members of the interdisciplinary team. Ultimately, functioning will be more accurately assessed to provide the highest quality of services to address the needs of the individual consumer of recreational therapy services.

To assist the developing RT professional, the text is arranged in chapters that introduce the reader to the foundations of assessment, the basics of the ICF, and the assessment of the consumer by diagnostic-related groups. Specific chapters will address evidence-based assessment for varying consumer groups, including older adults, mental health consumers, individuals with intellectual disabilities, and persons with physical disabilities, as well as the impacts of cultural awareness on service delivery. It is important for the developing professional to recognize that, although there are multiple examples of assessment by diagnostic-related group (DRG) or setting, functional limitations are not diagnosis specific and every consumer group will share similar functional needs and similar tools for measuring functional capacity.

Each author used the ICF model to provide insights into the multiple methods required to understand the person in relation to the ICF domains of Body Structure, Body Function, Activities and Participation, and the Environment. The text recognizes that active engagement in the community is the ultimate goal of all rehabilitation disciplines. Most chapters include case examples and review questions to promote student understanding of the ICF and the assessment process.

We trust you will find this journey in consumer assessment valuable as you prepare to deliver services to a diversity of individuals within the habilitation, rehabilitation, and preventative care settings. The following offers a brief summary of each chapter.

Chapter 1: The Complexities of Assessment and RT Service Delivery by King, Singleton, Skalko, and Hopper

This chapter introduces the Comprehensive Recreational Therapy Service Delivery model (CRTSD). The model illustrates how assessment and service delivery are interconnected and that recreational therapy assessment and service delivery are multifaceted. The CRTSD model integrates assessment, consumer rapport, activity analysis, and the utilization of the ICF for more effective and holistic service delivery. Using the CRTSD model as a conceptual view of the TR process, the chapter provides the

foundation for how the ICF teaches recreational therapy professionals to build an understanding of the person's ability based upon multiple inputs. The recognition of strengths, weaknesses, opportunities, and challenges are the key to understanding the abilities and capacity of the person. The chapter addresses what a recreational therapist should know about the use of tools and how they will facilitate or impede the process when working with specific consumer groups. This chapter also introduces an understanding that assessment is complex and that tools are only one component of the assessment process, as illustrated within the ICF.

Chapter 2: Principles of Assessment by Skalko, King, and Hopper

This chapter offers the reader a foundational perspective of assessment and key principles of the assessment process. It provides concepts about the assessment process and emphasizes the need for comprehensive approaches to assessment. Included are knowledge of psychometric properties of tests and measurements and a discussion on the use of valid and reliable assessment instruments. Also addressed are the challenges of securing and using evidence-based assessment instruments in recreational therapy practice. The chapter includes considerations for consumer interviewing and observation as necessary elements in the assessment process. As noted throughout the text, assessment is a focused, deliberate process, using valid and reliable means to determine the treatment needs of the consumers we serve.

Chapter 3: Understanding the *International Classification for Functioning, Disability and Health* (ICF) and Consumer Assessment by Skalko

The *International Classification of Functioning, Disability and Health* (ICF) places the individual in social and cultural context to examine the interactions of health and social conditions on a person with a disability through a biopsychosocial model. The ICF model provides insights into the complexities of consumer assessment through community participation (learning and applying knowledge, mobility, major life areas, etc.), physical factors (body functions and structure), and contextual factors (environmental, personal) of the person within society (WHO, 2001, p. 18). The ICF focuses on how people live with health conditions and how functioning can be enhanced for the person so they can lead a productive life. The indicators used within the ICF have implications for health care providers and policy makers in relation to the rights of individuals and groups.

The author offers an understanding of the ICF model and its connection to the assessment process. Of particular value is understanding how the ICF classification system can aid and affirm assessment goals and outcomes and coincides with the outcomes of the interdisciplinary treatment team.

Chapter 4: Documentation of Health Outcomes in Recreational Therapy by Loy and Skalko

Documentation is an essential skill for all practicing health care professionals. This chapter offers the reader key information regarding the documentation process. The chapter reviews the regulatory requirements and the profession's standards of practice related to documentation. In addition, the chapter offers key guidelines for documentation and reviews the dominant formats for documenting client progress in the APIE process. It is important to note that documentation is an essential function; it is not one of the processes of APIE but is nonetheless an essential activity in each phase of the process.

Chapter 4 also connects documentation to the *International Classification for Functioning, Disability and Health* (ICF) and to the use of SMART goals for treatment planning (Specific, Measurable, Attainable, Realistic, and Time limited). The chapter and associated appendix offer the student a primer on key medical abbreviations used in the documentation action.

Chapters 5 through 9 apply concepts of cultural competence and sensitivity in the assessment process, the assessment of older adults, behavioral health consumers, persons with intellectual and developmental impairments, and individuals with physically disabling conditions. Each chapter connects the assessment process with the application of the ICF to promote greater integration of the recreational therapy professional and the interdisciplinary team.

Chapter 5: Assessment and Aging: Considerations and Recommendations for Recreational Therapy by Janke and Van Puymbroeck

In chapter 5, the authors help the reader understand the unique aspects of an assessment process with older adults. Factors such as physical limitations (hearing loss, orthostatic hypotension), medications, and test environments are addressed to emphasize considerations needed when assessing older adults. Age-related considerations are also included to sensitize the recreational therapist to the broad range of variables that come into play when assessing the older adult consumer.

The chapter offers specific information on evidence-based assessment instruments for practice. As with all population-specific chapters, a case study for applying knowledge and principles of assessment and the ICF is included.

Chapter 6: Assessment and Behavioral Health by McCormick and Snethen

McCormick and Snethen bring to the forefront a transdiagnostic perspective to the assessment process. Congruent with the ICF, the transdiagnostic approach places less importance on the specific diagnosis and emphasizes addressing the maintenance of processes that promote dysfunction. The authors offer examples of how the transdiagnostic process relates to the ICF and how the professional might consider integrating the ICF classification system and Core Sets of functional areas for persons receiving mental health services into the assessment process.

Chapter 7: Assessment of Outcomes in Physical Disability: Considerations and Recommendations for Recreational Therapy by Loy

Loy provides a strong piece on understanding the comprehensive nature of assessment and persons with physically disabling conditions. Key concepts of assessment and the competencies needed in practice are presented.

Individual attributes that affect the assessment process, such as physical limitations and the varying abilities of the individual, are discussed. In addition, cognitive and communication limitations of persons with physically disabling conditions are presented to emphasize the complex nature of the assessment process for persons served in the physical rehabilitation setting.

Functional domains of vision, hearing, and balance are addressed, with examples of specific screening and assessment tools included in the chapter. In particular, the chapter addresses the issues of balance and the measurement of balance for persons receiving rehabilitation services. Other areas addressed by the author include pain, cardiovascular functioning, and neuromuscular and motor-related functions.

In the chapter, the author included means for assessing consumer activities and participation, including motor functioning measures to promote engagement in activities in the community. Assessments for individual mobility, fine motor manipulation, and wheelchair mobility are included. Information on the Functional Independence Measure (FIM), Leisure Competence Measures (LCM), Craig Handicap Assessment and Reporting Technique (CHART), and Community Integration Questionnaire (CIQ) provide direct information on a host of assessment instruments for use in settings that serve persons with physically disabling conditions.

Chapter 8: Recreational Therapy Assessment and Individuals With Intellectual Disabilities by Green and Jacobs

Green and Jacobs take the reader through an understanding of Intellectual Disability (ID) and the assessment process. The authors provide an understanding of the criteria used in the diagnostic process of Intellectual Disability including the criteria of intellectual functioning, adaptive behavior, and developmental period. The authors make the connection between the ICF and the diagnostic and assessment processes.

The chapter integrates the assessment process with the components of the ICF including *Body Structure and Function*, *Activities and Participation*, and *Environment*. Concepts of full engagement in the life of the community and factors that impact engagement in the life of the community are addressed. Issues such as social role validation and inclusion are discussed, including the varied levels of participation by individuals with intellectual disabilities in the life of the community. The assessment of environmental factors in order to address the needs of individuals with ID are also introduced.

Chapter 9: Assessing Clients With Diverse Cultural Backgrounds by Nagata, Hopper, and Zaremski

To effectively and appropriately engage in the assessment of any individual, an understanding and sensitivity to the individual's culture is paramount. This chapter addresses the changing multicultural nature of the world's population.

To develop a more complete understanding of culture, the authors address a range of factors that affect assessment and cultural awareness. Issues such as social dominance, ethnocentrism, individualism and collectivism, and cultural assimilation and ethnic identity provide the reader a more complete picture of the challenges for individuals from diverse cultures.

Key concepts of culture as they relate to the assessment process are also discussed, including the impacts of language and meaning on assessment inquiries. This chapter brings to the forefront the need for recreational therapy professionals to increase their own understanding of and attention to cultural competence and sensitivity in the assessment process.

Chapter 10: Final Reflections by Skalko and Singleton

The last chapter of the text provides a summation of the key concepts within the text. Utilizing the Comprehensive Recreational Therapy Service Delivery model in conjunction with the ICF integrates key recreational therapy strategies, the ICF, and the assessment process.

We trust you will find that each chapter develops your knowledge, skills, and abilities in the assessment process and its connection to the *International Classification for Functioning, Disability and Health*. Students and practitioners will find foundational knowledge on the ICF, consumer assessment, and the complex nature of assessment useful when serving the public. Assessment is a complex task regardless of setting, and it is incumbent on the practitioner to attend to the complexities of individual client assessment. Each chapter brings to light the underlying concepts of assessment by population and the interrelatedness of the assessment process and the ICF. Case studies, discussion questions, and learning activities are included throughout in order to facilitate the readers' competencies in recreational therapy assessment.

REFERENCES

Austin, D.R. (1991). *Therapeutic recreation: Processes and techniques* (2nd ed.). Champaign, IL: Sagamore.

King, A. (2014). *The pick of the litter? Understanding standardized assessment tools and the assessment process with older adults in therapeutic recreation practitioners* (Master's thesis). Dalhousie University, Halifax.

O'Morrow, G.S., & Reynolds, R.P. (1989). *Therapeutic recreation: A helping profession*. Englewood Cliffs, NJ: Prentice Hall.

Peterson, C.A., & Stumbo, N.J. (2009). Client assessment. In N.J. Stumbo & C.A. Peterson (Eds.), *Therapeutic recreation program design* (5th ed., pp. 249-298). San Francisco, CA: Pearson.

World Health Organization. (2001). *International classification of functioning, disability and health*. Geneva, Switzerland: Author.

CHAPTER 1

The Complexities of Assessment and RT Service Delivery

Andrea King, MA, CTRS • Jerome F. Singleton, PhD, CTRS
Thomas K. Skalko, PhD, LRT/CTRS, FDRT • Tristan Hopper, PhD, CTRS

LEARNING OBJECTIVES

Upon completion of the text, the student will demonstrate:

- Knowledge of RT service delivery models and practice settings.
- Knowledge of the APIE process (assessment, planning, implementation, and evaluation).
- Knowledge of the scope of practice of recreational therapy for program planning.
- Knowledge of the systems approach to program planning and service delivery.
- Knowledge of principles underlying the therapeutic process, with emphasis on interaction between the RT professional and the client.
- Knowledge of the role of the recreational therapist as a member of the interdisciplinary treatment team.
- Knowledge of the Comprehensive Recreational Therapy Service Delivery (CRTSD) model.

Therapeutic recreation (TR) involves the Assess, Plan, Implement, and Evaluate (APIE) process. This process allows the therapist to systematically develop a program based on the person's abilities. Assessment is a complex process using multiple inputs to ensure we understand the functional abilities of the consumer (ATRA, 2013; King, 2014; WHO, 2001). The planning, implementation, and evaluation then builds on this understanding. Assessment processes can look very different based on which diagnostic group of clients you are working with, resources available to the practitioner, and the influence of other practitioners. What is most important to remember is that assessment is a process, not a one-time event (Stumbo & Peterson, 2003). Common means of gathering information for assessments include

- medical history review;
- consultation with other health care team members (Anderson & Heyne, 2012; Austin, 1998; Smale & Gillies, 2012; Stumbo & Peterson, 2003);
- the administration of a valid and reliable assessment instrument for the condition, population, or area in which the practitioner requires insight (Burlingame & Blaschko, 2002);
- interviews with the client or family;
- observations; and
- evaluation of resources in the community.

We reside in a global village. Individuals are migrating from developing countries to developed countries (MacNeil & Gould, 2012), bringing their cultural values and personal perspectives. RT service providers need to understand how these individuals frame their lived experience. Intersectionality theory (Crenshaw, 1991) provides a framework to understand what an RT practitioner should consider when working with people across the life course. Intersectionality is the idea that disadvantages in life are not rooted in a single factor, but rather are the consequences

of multiple factors (Hankivsky, 2014) (see chapter 9).

This chapter will provide insights into how the various RT perspectives have emerged to structure RT service, how some RT practitioners identified what they perceived to be the information they need to understand the person's abilities, and how the *International Classification of Functioning, Disability and Health* (ICF) provides a consistent process for classifying information for RT practitioners.

Perspectives

Therapeutic recreation is a profession that empowers the individual's abilities to engage in a meaningful experience. To assist RT professionals in understanding people's abilities, scholars have developed various perspectives to understand how the RT process is transferred to practice.

The various perspectives that have emerged within the therapeutic recreation profession, such as Therapeutic Recreation: A Continuum (Frye & Peters, 1972), Leisure Ability (Peterson & Gunn, 1984; Stumbo & Peterson, 2003), Health Protection/Health Promotion (Austin, 1998), Strength Based Approach (Anderson & Heyne, 2012), and Optimizing Lifelong Health and Well-Being: A Health Enhancing Model of Therapeutic Recreation (Wilhite, Keller, & Caldwell, 1999), are often taught within professional preparation programs. However, it is the practitioner that attempts to define their services within the framework in which they were introduced.

These models are scholars' perceptions of how the RT process (APIE) would be transferred to practice within the framework proposed. The terms used in each of the models reflect the conceptual frameworks of the authors who developed the framework. The question arises: How do practitioners view the process they use to understand the delivery of RT service? What conceptual model could RT practitioners use in practice? What information do the RT practitioners use to empower the people with whom they work?

Comprehensive Recreational Therapy Service Delivery (CRTSD) Model

King (2014) explored how Certified Therapeutic Recreation Specialists (CTRS) working with older adults conducted their assessments and the implications of assessment on their practice. The research led to the development of the Comprehensive Recreational Therapy Service Delivery (CRTSD) model by King, Singleton, and Skalko that is presented in this text.

King (2014), upon identifying themes that emerged during her study from RT (CTRS) practitioners who worked with older adults, framed the basis of the Comprehensive Recreational Therapy Service Delivery model for discussion. The model demonstrates the complexities of the assessment process through delivery (figure 1.1). The CRTSD model also illustrates the complexity of assessment within the RT process (i.e., Assess, Plan, Implement, and Evaluate).

The CRTSD model encompasses traditional RT assessment processes (e.g., assessment of specific behavioral and emotional areas, medical review, observation, interview with client or family). The model also provides insights

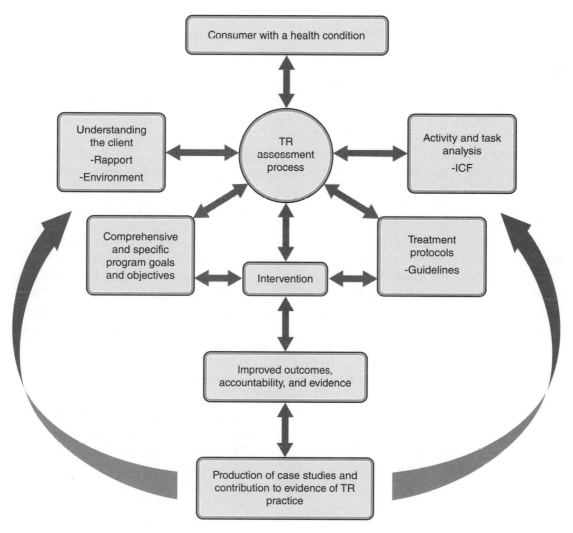

FIGURE 1.1 Comprehensive Recreational Therapy Service Delivery model.
King, Singleton, and Skalko, 2018

into the external factors that practitioners can use not only to inform their assessment process but to guide their practice. Assessment of each client should reflect the purpose of the service delivery (in keeping with what you provide as a service) and ways that service delivery can inform or guide how we treat clients. In the study, King (2014) found that not all RT practitioners connect activity or task analysis to the assessment process. Activity analysis and task analysis provide insights into the complexities of the experience and identify areas needed to be addressed to assist the client to reach their ability level.

Activity Analysis

The utilization of activity analysis and task analysis allows the therapist to evaluate the demands of an activity and to break down the activity into discrete tasks for successful engagement. According to the ICF, an activity "is the execution of a task or action by an individual" (WHO, 2001, p. 17). Every activity can be analyzed (activity analysis) (Avedon, 1974; Avedon & Sutton-Smith, 1971; Stumbo & Peterson, 2003; Wehman & Schleien, 1981) to determine the physical, cognitive, affective, and social demands of the activity to evaluate whether the consumer can successfully engage in the activity. In addition, administrative demands of an activity must also be analyzed.

Activity analysis requires that the RT professional break an activity into component parts. Stumbo and Peterson (2003, p. 181) outlined the following principles of activity analysis:

- Analyze the activity as it is normally engaged in.
- Rate the activity as compared to all other activities.
- Analyze the activity without regard for any specific disability group.
- Analyze the activity with regard to the minimal level of skills required for basic successful participation.

Stumbo and Peterson (2003, pp. 181–184) also provide an activity analysis form that covers physical, social, cognitive, affective, and administrative aspects required for an activity.

From a physical domain perspective, the therapist must determine (based on an assessment of the consumer) whether the consumer has the physical skills (competencies) to successfully participate in an activity or task. This will include fine motor skills, gross motor skills, cardiovascular fitness, coordination, and other physical functioning aspects. If the person cannot perform a task or activity in one or more areas of the physical domain, then the therapist must assist the individual in developing the physical skills (e.g., grasping a paint brush or ambulating on different surfaces) necessary for successful engagement.

When addressing the cognitive domain, the therapist must determine whether the individual has the cognitive capacity or knowledge to engage in the activity. Some activities require complex rules or the memorization of materials to successfully engage. An assessment of the individual's cognitive abilities is in order. This assessment may be performed by the agency's psychology staff and supplemented with observational assessments of any number of treatment team members.

Next, the therapist must determine whether the individual possesses the social skills for successful engagement in the activity. For instance, does the individual have the skills to interact in one-on-one situations, small group, or large group activities? Does the consumer possess the social skills for establishing and maintaining interpersonal relationships? Again, via an analysis of the social demands of the activity, an assessment of the individual's social skills will allow for a determination of their ability to engage in a particular activity (Avedon, 1974).

For the social components to the experience, Stumbo and Peterson (2003) used Avedon's (1974) classification system of interaction patterns found in recreation activities to expand on the social aspects required. These patterns are shown in table 1.1.

Finally, activities must also be analyzed to determine their administrative demands. Is the activity feasible? It may not be administratively feasible to utilize aquatic rehabilitation activ-

TABLE 1.1   Characteristics of Interaction Patterns

Interaction pattern	Characteristics
Intraindividual	An action taking place within the mind of a person or involving the mind and part of the body, but requiring no contact with another person or an external object
Extraindividual	Activity directed by a person toward an object in the environment requiring no contact with another person
Aggregate	Action directed by a person toward an object in the environment while in the company of other persons who are also directing action toward objects in the environment; action is not directed toward one another, and no interaction among participants is required or necessary
Interindividual	Action of a competitive nature directed by one person toward another
Unilateral	Action of a competitive nature among three or more persons, one of whom is an antagonist, or "it"
Intragroup	Action of a cooperative nature by two or more persons intent upon reaching a mutual goal; action requires positive verbal and nonverbal interaction
Intergroup	Action of a competitive nature between two or more intragroups
Multilateral	Action of a competitive nature among three or more persons, with no one person as an antagonist

ities if the building and operations of a pool are beyond the capacity of the organization. The same may hold true for such activities as hippotherapy. Even more simple activities such as an overnight camping can have significant administrative demands, including staffing, staff overtime, and cost. The scope and outcomes of service delivery must be congruent with the mission of the agency.

Wehman and Schleien (1981) provide an in-depth analysis for leisure skills assessment in their text. They discuss the *Evaluating Leisure Skills Assessment Guide, Behavioral Variables for Leisure Assessment*, and a model for selection of leisure skills. They build upon the identification of the client's interests by identifying how the task should be broken into component parts that are measurable. This process parallels the task of writing measurable objectives (Wehman & Schleien, 1981).

Every activity has a set of demands (knowledge, skills, and abilities) to successfully engage in the activity. It is the recreational therapist's responsibility to assess these domains for an accurate evaluation of the person's functional skills for engagement.

Task Analysis

The utilization of task analysis allows the therapist to break down any activity into discrete tasks, much like the ICF. Every activity encompasses a set of discrete tasks (what the ICF refers to as activities) in order to engage. Painting, for instance, requires grasping a brush, mixing paints, applying paints to a canvas, and cleaning brushes. While this is a broad description, the tasks involved in painting are rather complex and beyond the scope of this text. The key, however, is for the therapist to systematically break down each activity in this way. Coupled with an assessment of the individual's abilities, the therapist can determine which tasks may be more challenging for the client and develop an intervention plan to develop the requisite skills for a given task.

From the assessment process and the application of task analysis for a given activity (as defined by the ICF), the therapist is able to identify specific program goals and SMART objectives (specific, measurable, achievable, relevant, and time limited). By utilizing discrete outcomes, the therapist can develop intervention strategies to improve the functional abilities of the individual. It is important to note that the therapist may be directly addressing the functional area or may be utilizing client strengths to compensate for a functional limitation. These assets may be individual or may be available through technologies.

Following the intervention, the therapist will engage in a reassessment of the consumer to evaluate progress. Too often, the entry-level therapist does not realize that through proper measurement, the application of an intervention or treatment protocol, and the evaluation of the results, the makings of a case study have been completed. Through the application and documentation of the comprehensive RT process, the evidence-based practice cycle is completed and the practitioner has the information for the publication of results.

Breaking activities down into steps will help delineate to the therapist where a client can functionally complete an activity or where the client may struggle. All of these methodologies help inform intervention selection and client performance; an evaluation of the implementation stage of the APIE process would provide

the recreational therapist with outcomes that could inform future assessment procedures and client interventions.

King's (2014) study provided insights into how some RT practitioners apply the APIE process in their service delivery. The CRTSD model illustrates the inputs the RT practitioners identified, during the study, that assisted them in understanding the abilities of the person receiving services. Information collected through formal assessment, activity analysis, understanding the client, rapport development, environment, and task analysis all provide information for the RT process. The inputs lead to the intervention based upon the person's abilities and interests, which leads to improved outcomes, accountability, and evidence. The role of activity and task analysis was not used by all therapists in the study due to the perceived complexities of the process. By understanding the physical, social, affective, cognitive, and administrative demands of an activity, the recreational therapist is better able to integrate the ICF classification system into their assessment practices and identify discrete outcomes for client improvement.

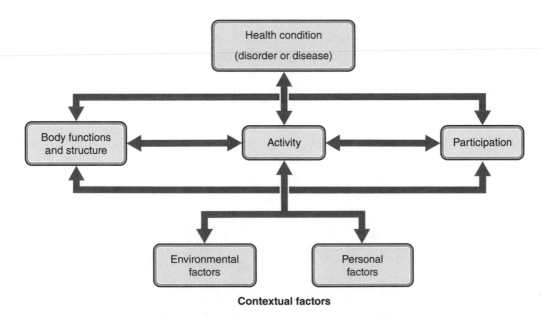

FIGURE 1.2   *International Classification of Functioning, Disability and Health* (ICF).

Reprinted by permission from *International Classification of Functioning, Disability and Health*, pg. 17, copyright 2001 (Geneva, World Health Organization).

International Classification of Functioning, Disability and Health (ICF)

The ICF works to classify functioning, including Body Structure, Body Function, Activities and Participation, and Environment (see figure 1.2).

The ICF model places the individual within their physical, social, environmental, and cultural context through a biopsychosocial model to examine the interactions of health and social conditions on a person with a disabling condition (WHO, 2001) (see chapter 3).

Summary

Like the ICF (WHO, 2001), the CRTSD model begins with a health condition. An assessment is completed to evaluate the impacts of the health condition on the physical, social, and cognitive functioning of the consumer. Note that areas of the assessment may be completed by varying members of the treatment team. The assessment will also include a range of other information to fully *understand the person* (e.g., family supports, technologies available, social networks, environmental challenges).

Assessment is the key to the APIE process. Assessment is as multidimensional as RT professionals. The CRTSD reflects assessment as a process and illustrates the interactivity of understanding the client, the role of comprehensive program planning (CPP) and specific program planning (SPP) in assessment, diagnostic protocol guidelines, and the role of activity analysis. This information frames the understanding of the person and guides the assessment process and the planning, implementation, and evaluation of services.

Since assessment is a multidimensional process and not a single instrument, the assessment process has interactive components that form how the RT professional understands the person and their abilities to engage in meaningful experiences. The CRTSD model integrates each aspect of the assessment process and service delivery (e.g., understanding the client

and their environment, diagnostic protocol guidelines, and activity analysis). The model addresses several elements of the assessment process, including the interactivity of each component on the assessment process and the realization that assessment is a process and not just the tools utilized. The tools, however, are also essential elements of the assessment process.

The CRTSD model, like the *International Classification of Functioning, Disability and Health* (ICF), is a dynamic perspective of service delivery where each element affects the overall outcome of services. Globally, the ICF model places the individual within their physical, social, environmental, and cultural context through a biopsychosocial model to examine the interactions of health and social conditions on a person with a disabling condition (WHO, 2001). The CRTSD also reflects the dynamic interactions within the APIE process as, like the ICF, a biopsychosocial model for service delivery.

The RT process (APIE) fits well with the ICF and recreational therapy practice. The foundation of the APIE process is the assessment phase. The assessment phase establishes the framework for planning the experience, implementing the experience, evaluating the experience, and documenting each phase of the process. Assessment also assists in the classification of the individual's functioning within the ICF.

Assessment involves understanding the person (e.g., abilities, condition, culture, gender, race), the activity (task analysis, activity analysis, cultural framework of experience), the assessment tools (reliability and validity), the RT process (APIE), and comprehensive and specific program planning. Understanding the complexities of the assessment process in context to comprehensive service delivery offers a foundation for the full integration of services in practice. It is essential to also understand the principles of consumer assessment and the multitude of factors to be considered when utilizing assessment instruments and processes.

REFLECTION QUESTIONS

1. Identify one of the perspectives promulgated within RT practice and offer an analysis.
2. How does the perspective you chose influence RT practice?
3. Identify at least three key elements of the Comprehensive Recreational Therapy Service Delivery model.
4. Explain how assessment is utilized within the CRTSD.

REFERENCES

American Therapeutic Recreation Association. (2013). *Standards for the practice of recreational therapy*. Hattiesburg, MS: Author.

Anderson, L., & Heyne, L.A. (2012). *Therapeutic recreation practice: A strengths approach*. Urbana, IL: Sagamore-Venture.

Austin, D.R. (1998). The health protection/health promotion model. *Therapeutic Recreation Journal, 32*(2), 109-117.

Avedon, E.M. (1974). *Therapeutic recreation service: An applied behavioral science approach*. Englewood Cliffs, NJ: Prentice Hall.

Avedon, E.M., & Sutton-Smith, B. (1971). *Study of games*. New York: Wiley.

Burlingame, J., & Blaschko, T.M. (2002). *Assessment tools for recreational therapy and related fields* (3rd ed.). Ravensdale, WA: Idyll Arbor.

Crenshaw, K. (1991). Mapping the margins: Intersectionality, identity politics, and violence against women of color. *Stanford Law Review, 43*(6), 1241-1299.

Frye, V., & Peters, M. (1972). *Therapeutic recreation: Its theory, philosophy, and practice*. Harrisburg, PA: Stackpole Books.

Hankivsky, O. (2014). *Intersectionality 101*. Burnaby, BC: The Institute for Intersectionality Research & Policy, Simon Fraser University. Retrieved from www.sfu.ca/iirp/documents/resources/101_Final.pdf

King, A. (2014). *The pick of the litter? Understanding standardized assessment tools and the assessment process with older adults in therapeutic recreation practitioners*. (Master's thesis). Dalhousie University, Halifax.

MacNeil, R.D., & Gould, D.L. (2012). Global perspectives on leisure and aging. In H. Gibson & J.F. Singleton (Eds.), *Leisure and aging: Theory to practice* (pp. 3-26). Champaign, IL: Human Kinetics.

Peterson, C., & Gunn, S.L. (1984). *Therapeutic recreation program design: Principles and practices* (2nd ed.). Englewood Cliffs, NJ: Prentice Hall.

Porter, H., & Van Puymbroeck, M. (2007). Utilization of the *International Classification of Functioning, Disability, and Health* within therapeutic recreation practice. *Therapeutic Recreation, 41*(1), 47-60.

Smale, B., & Gillies, J. (2012). Studying leisure in the context of aging. In H. Gibson & J.F. Singleton (Eds.), *Leisure and aging: Theory to practice* (pp. 67-94). Champaign, IL: Human Kinetics.

Stumbo, N., & Peterson, C.A. (2003). *Therapeutic recreation program design* (4th ed.). Boston, MA: Allyn & Bacon.

Wehman, P., & Schleien, S.J. (1981). *Leisure programs for handicapped persons: Adaptations, techniques and curriculum*. Baltimore, MD: University Park Press.

Wilhite, B., Keller, J., & Caldwell, L. (1999). Optimizing lifelong health and well-being: A health enhancing model of therapeutic recreation. *Therapeutic Recreation Journal, 33*, 98-108.

World Health Organization. (2001). *International Classification of Functioning, Disability and Health*. Geneva, Switzerland: Author.

ADDITIONAL RESOURCES

Howard, D., Browning, C., & Lee, Y. (2007). *The International Classification of Functioning, Disability and Health*: Therapeutic recreation code sets and salient diagnostic code sets. *Therapeutic Recreation Journal, 41*(1), 60-81.

Howard, D., Russoniello, C., & Rogers, D. (2004). Healthy People 2010 and therapeutic recreation: Professional opportunities promote public health. *Therapeutic Recreation Journal, 28*(2), 116-132.

Hutchison, P., & McGill, J. (1992). *Leisure, integration, and community.* Toronto: Leisurability.

National Council for Therapeutic Recreation Certification. (2018). About recreational therapy. Retrieved January 8, 2018, from https://nctrc.org/about-ncrtc/about-recreational-therapy

Schleien, S.J. (1993). Access and inclusion in community services. *Parks and Recreation, 28*(4), 66-72.

Schleien, S.J., Germ, P.A., & McAvoy, L.H. (1996). Inclusive community leisure services: Recommended professional practices and barriers encountered. *Therapeutic Recreation Journal, 30*, 260-273.

Schleien, S.J., Light, C.L., McAvoy, L.H., & Baldwin, C.K. (1989). Best professional practices: Serving persons with severe multiple disabilities. *Therapeutic Recreation Journal, 23*(3), 27-40.

Schleien, S.J., McAvoy, L.H., Lais, G.J., & Rynders, J.E. (1993). *Integrated outdoor education and adventure programs.* Champaign, IL: Sagamore Publishing.

Schleien, S.J., Porter, J., & Wehman, P. (1979). An assessment of leisure skill needs of developmentally disabled individuals. *Therapeutic Recreation Journal, 13*(3), 16-21.

CHAPTER 2

Principles of Assessment

Thomas K. Skalko, PhD, LRT/CTRS, FDRT • Andrea King, MA, CTRS

Tristan Hopper, PhD, CTRS

CHAPTER OBJECTIVES

Upon completion of the text, the student will demonstrate:

- Knowledge of psychometric properties of tests and measurements.
- Knowledge of evidence-based recreational therapy assessment instruments used to determine physical, cognitive, emotional, and social functioning of clients.
- Knowledge of the World Health Organization's (WHO) *International Classification of Functioning, Disability and Health* (ICF) as a method of assessing individual functioning and the impact of activity limitations and restrictions to participation in life activities, independence, satisfaction, and quality of life.
- Knowledge of interviewing stages and strategies.
- Skill in applying ICF functional domains to client assessment.

This chapter will introduce the reader to the basic aspects of assessment and the assessment process. As noted in chapter 1, assessment is a complex process. It is therefore important to recognize that assessment is a multifaceted action that requires an understanding of principles necessary for valid and reliable outcomes. This chapter will introduce the reader to what assessment is and its role in the recreational therapy standards of practice. Considerations of what the recreational therapist should think about when selecting an assessment instrument are addressed. As with any concept, client assessment has both strengths and limitations. It is incumbent upon the therapist to understand the strengths and limitations of any assessment instrument and process and to integrate modifications as appropriate. In addition, assessment as it relates to the *International Classification of Functioning, Disability and Health* (ICF) are introduced.

What Is Assessment?

In the context of recreational therapy practice, assessment is a systematic process for collecting valid and reliable information on the functional performance of an individual. This would include both the individual's functional limitations and strengths. As noted in the *Standards for the Practice of Recreational Therapy* (ATRA, 2013, p. 15),

> The recreational therapist receives and responds, consistent with standards, regulatory requirements and policies for the setting, to requests, including referrals and physician orders, for assessment and treatment; and conducts an individualized assessment to collect systematic, comprehensive and accurate data necessary to determine a course of action and subsequent individualized treatment plan.

In turn, it is the obligation of the recreational therapist to complete an assessment of the individual that provides valid, reliable, and meaningful results in order to deliver quality intervention services. These services may include a full range of strategies from education to structured activities in order to improve the functional limitations of the consumer. Actions may also include activities and services that complement the individual's strengths as a means to compensate for any limitations. Ultimately, recreational therapy and all rehabilitation services should promote the individual's active engagement in the life of the community.

To accomplish the outcome of optimal functioning and engagement, it is important for the therapist to understand the characteristics of sound assessment in order to focus service delivery to meet the needs of the consumer. This chapter will present basic information of the principles of assessment, including the elements of validity and reliability. While it is unlikely the entry-level therapist will be engaged in the process of completing validity and reliability studies on assessment instruments, it is important to be able to read existing information on an instrument and to determine whether it is appropriate for their setting and population.

Validity and Reliability: What Are They? Why Are They Important?

As a recreational therapist or a student, the overriding question is whether the assessment tools used are in fact measuring what you intend them to measure. Importantly, understanding the concepts of assessment *validity* and *reliability* is essential. Figure 2.1 offers an excellent representation of both concepts (Trochim, 2018).

As depicted in figure 2.1, an instrument may be (1) reliable but not valid (it consistently measures a variable but the measurement is not accurate), (2) valid but not reliable (it measures the variable but it is not consistent in measurement), (3) neither valid nor reliable (it neither measures the variable accurately nor is it consistent), or (4) both valid and reliable (it consistently and accurately measures the variable in question). Another way to think about it is like using a bathroom scale. If the scale consistently measures you at a given weight each time you step on it in a given period of

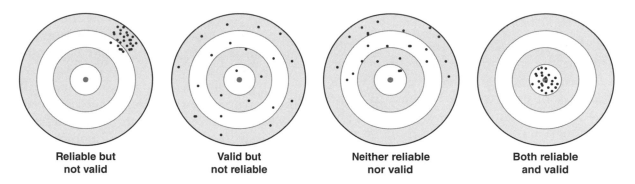

Reliable but not valid   **Valid but not reliable**   **Neither reliable nor valid**   **Both reliable and valid**

FIGURE 2.1   The relationship between reliability and validity.

Reprinted by permission from W. Trochim, *Research Methods Knowledge Base*, Web (Fairfax, VA: Center for Social Science Research, 2018).

time, it is reliable. The question, however, is whether the scale accurately measures your weight—so don't be fooled by scales that give you false low weight readings. If it measures accurately, it is a valid instrument to measure your weight.

Assessment Validity

For outcome measures such as surveys or tests, *validity* refers to the accuracy of measurement results. Here validity refers to how well the results of the assessment tool actually reflect the underlying outcomes of interest (Sullivan, 2011, p. 1). It is important to note that validity is not a property of the tool but more of the interpretation of the results with a specific population or individual. Simply, *validity* refers to the degree to which the results of your assessment tool measure what is intended. So, "validity refers to the *accuracy* of measurement" (Sullivan, 2011, p. 1).

To determine the validity of assessment tools, it is important to first understand what you are trying to measure. Secondly, it is important for the recreational therapist to be able to determine whether a selected instrument meets the criteria for validity. The therapist should have a basic understanding of the types of validity, including face validity, content validity, criterion-related validity, and construct validity, among other approaches. Establishing or determining validity is like constructing an evidence-based position on how well a tool measures what it is supposed to measure. Support may be identified in the

instrument content, response process, relationships with other variables, and outcomes (Sullivan, 2011). The recreational therapist should understand how the forms of validity differ from one another but is not likely to be engaged in a validation study for an instrument.

Face Validity

In face validity, the practitioner (or researcher) would perform a general evaluation of the operationalization of the instrument and determine, "on its face," whether the instrument subjectively appears to be a good reflection of the construct or variable being measured. Individuals would express whether they believe the instrument measures its intent—that it measures what it is intended to measure. If the intent is clear to a member of the general population, it is said to have high face validity. For example, on an instrument to measure self-esteem, the respondent might be asked if an item "I feel good about myself" would reflect self-esteem. The respondent may agree that this is a function of self-esteem. On the other hand, "I think global warming is a myth" as an item would have little face validity in an instrument measuring self-esteem. Another example may be an item on a test measuring depression. A statement that says, "Recently, I don't feel very good about myself" may reflect a state of depression. The problem with such instruments, however, is that a respondent can manipulate the answers to reflect a different state of emotion. Face validity is the weakest means for establishing the validity of an instrument.

Content Validity

In evaluating assessment instruments and processes, the practitioner needs to critique the content of the instrument (content validity). A jury of experts may be used to make a professional judgment as to whether the instrument potentially measures the content or the operationalization of a variable. A simple example of content validity would be a test to measure math concepts like the addition of single numbers. Does the test content accurately reflect adding single digit numbers? If the content included multiplication, it would not be appropriate for the first grader learning to add single digit numbers. Therefore, a jury of experts could determine that these items would not be valid for the evaluation instrument.

In practice, the therapist may want to assess knowledge and practices of a healthy lifestyle as an outcome of a lifestyle awareness group. The assessment instrument may measure knowledge and individual practice in each of the modules of the program, including such elements as healthy eating habits, physical activity and exercise, and stress management. In turn, the therapist could determine the level of the consumer's knowledge in each of these areas and what the consumer's practices included. Therefore, the assessment would include items that would reflect the outcomes of the designed intervention strategy in each of the lifestyle content areas and what the consumer's lifestyle reflected. The designed instrument could then be evaluated by a jury of experts to determine whether the content of the assessment instrument possessed content validity in each of the areas covered under lifestyle awareness program. Items of the assessment instrument could then be evaluated for inclusion or exclusion. The assessment would allow the therapist to determine an individual's current knowledge base on a given construct or subject area and a reflection of current lifestyle habits.

Criterion-Related Validity

Criterion-related validity may include concurrent or predictive validity. Simply put, in concurrent criteria-related validity, the therapist or researcher would check the outcome of a longer version of an instrument concurrently with a new, shorter assessment instrument. If an instrument on quality of life was 90 items long, it is more likely many of the respondents may experience test fatigue and not complete the instrument or randomly pick answers to get through the assessment. Through a series of comparisons between the original instrument and the shorter version, the therapist could then determine whether the shorter instrument could provide a statistically comparable and valid outcome score. So, in concurrent validity, the assessment instrument is compared to an already established instrument measuring the construct or variable. From a practical application perspective, a new assessment instrument (25 items) that measures quality of life may be compared to an existing instrument (90 items). If the interpretation of the results is statistically the same, the instruments may possess concurrent validity and it may be more efficient to use the shorter instrument for similar results.

The second form of criterion-related validity is predictive validity. In simple terms, predictive validity establishes that the score on a particular instrument can make an accurate prediction of future performance in a given area (e.g., intelligence, honesty, depression) (McLeod, 2013). The predictions are theory based and represent how the interpretation of scores from the instrument can predict future performance on the variable of interest. Because performance is variable, relationships among high, medium, and low scores should be consistent. An example may be the use of an intelligence assessment as a predictor of cognitive performance in older adulthood.

Construct Validity

Construct validity approximates the assertion that the operationalization of a variable accurately reflects its construct (Sullivan, 2011). Construct validity requires a strong and sound operationalization of what is being measured. Constructs like self-esteem, attitude, self-concept, and IQ all require a means of reflecting the concept and determining whether the interpretation of the results of the instrument adequately reflect the construct in question. As noted by Richter and Werner (2015), "Constructs may have one (unidimensional) or more than one (multidimensional) domain. For example, health-related quality of life is a multidimensional construct conceptualized to have multiple domains including social function, physical function, and psychological function" (p. 150).

Ultimately, the therapist is not likely to perform tests for validity but will want to know the validity of an instrument from the test developer. If the developer has not established the validity of an assessment instrument, the interpretation of results will be suspect. When exploring the adoption and use of an assessment instrument, the therapist can seek published articles on the validity and reliability of a given instrument. Additional information can be obtained from the publisher of a given instrument as a means to evaluate its appropriateness for the setting and population of interest. Finally, there are multiple electronic resources for seeking information on assessment instruments (e.g., www.sralab. org/rehabilitation-measures). As a resource, the Rehabilitation Measures site offers some comprehensive information of instruments, including their validity and reliability.

Assessment Reliability

Assessment reliability refers to the consistency of assessment results. In other words, reliability indicates the dependability or consistency of

the assessment tool. Reliability ensures that if a therapist were to administer the same assessment tool to the same subject, the results received will be statistically the same. Additionally, if a therapist and second therapist were to administer the same assessment, the results should be very similar. It is important for the recreational therapist to understand that reliability of an assessment tool does not mean that it is reliable for all population groups, and this should be considered before using a standardized tool with a specific population group.

Reliability of an instrument can be established in numerous ways. The following offers a simple review of the processes used in determining reliability. It is important to note that these approaches are used to test the reliability of an instrument for assessment and for research purposes. Cook and Beckman (2006) offer a good discussion on determining the reliability of assessment instruments. Table 2.1 offers a summary for determining reliability.

Test-Retest Reliability

Test-retest reliability involves administering a test or assessment to a group of subjects and following up with a readministration of the test at a later date. The key is to not give the retest too soon as respondents may recall their previous answers. However, if the administration between tests is too long, the difference in results may be from other factors. Typically,

TABLE 2.1 Types of Reliability Testing

Test	Method	Analyses
Test-retest	Uses administration and readministration of the assessment to the same subject(s) at a different time	Pearson's *r* correlation
Interrater reliability	Uses concurrent administration by different raters to determine level of agreement on a measured construct	Percentage of rater agreement
Internal consistency	Determines whether the items in an instrument consistently measure the same construct vs. other constructs	Split-half reliability Chronbach's Alpha Kuder-Richardson
Parallel forms	Uses two versions of the same instrument	Pearson's *r* correlation

Summarized from Cook & Beckman (2006).

a Pearson r analysis on the test results will determine the correlation of the two attempts. A correlation of $r = .93$ would reflect a high correlation between the two administrations and therefore reflect a high level of reliability.

For example, if you were interested in assessing a person's quality of life, you could administer a quality of life assessment. Following a reasonable period of time, you could readminister the assessment and determine the reliability of the assessment instrument.

The same approach may be used in the measurement of state and trait anxiety. However, while a person's trait anxiety may not show much variability in scoring, a person's state anxiety is very susceptible to the moment in time and may very well reflect considerable variability.

Interrater Reliability

Interrater reliability occurs when different raters assess the same construct at the same time. If the construct or behavior is well defined, then there should be consistency between the scores or measures. The higher the percentage of agreement on the scoring of the assessment, the higher the interrater reliability. So, an interrater reliability of .85 indicates that there is an 85 percent agreement on the scoring of the individual on the defined construct or behavior. For instance, as noted by Podsiadlo and Richardson (1991), the Timed Up and Go Test for balance has strong interrater reliability and it also has strong reliability with other scales like the scores on the Berg Balance Scale ($r = -0.81$). When utilizing the many forms of assessment, training and experience lead to more consistent results.

To establish the internal consistency of an assessment instrument, a split-half reliability method may be applied. The split-half method measures the extent to which different halves of an assessment contribute to the construct being measured. In the split-half method, an assessment is administered and the results of separate halves are compared. The method may compare the results of the first half of the assessment with the results of the second half of the assessment, or it could compare even items with odd items on the assessment. A statistical analysis (e.g., Chronbach's Alpha, Kuder-Richardson) would determine whether individual items are reliable. If the reliability of an item is low ($r = .15$) then the item would warrant removal because it is not reliable. This approach is most valuable with large assessment instruments in order to remove items with low reliability (McLeod, 2013).

A basic understanding of these concepts is essential in understanding the validity and reliability of assessment instruments. In order for a recreational therapist or student to determine whether an instrument should be utilized, it is essential that they understand what both validity and reliability mean and how these concepts are measured.

Accessing Assessment Tools

Being able to locate and access assessment tools is key to utilizing valid and reliable assessment instruments. Generally, assessment tools are available through the developer of the tool, through published literature, or through numerous online resources. This may pose challenges for some practitioners who are unaware of available resources.

Throughout the text, efforts were made to include references and access to a host of valid and reliable instruments. Organized by diagnostic-related groups, these resources offer the practitioner access to information for use in assessing and delivering services to the consumer. Many of the identified instruments in the various chapters have common themes or functional variables being measured. The therapist should also not shy away from seeking agency support to purchase an appropriate assessment tool for their practice.

There are additional aspects of client assessment that the therapist must consider. These aspects include the development of requisite skills for effective interviewing as an element of the assessment process. In addition, the therapist must develop strong skills in client observation for consistent assessment outcomes.

Understanding Interviewing Principles in the Assessment Process

Often the assessment process begins with an interview with the consumer. The interview offers insights about the person but does not always offer valid and reliable information about the individual's functional capacity or other measures for treatment planning by the recreational therapist. The interview does, however, provide invaluable information that will assist in the treatment planning process and direct the collection of additional information on the person's perceived limitations and strengths.

Brédart, Marrel, Abetz-Webb, Lasch, and Acquadro (2014) offer some insights for patient-centered interviewing. Initially, the therapist must determine the depth of the interview, how standardized the interview should be, and how much control, as an interviewer, they choose to exercise. There are multiple ways to conduct an interview. The therapist must utilize an appropriate approach for the individual consumer and one that complements their individual style. If you are generating quantitative information, the interview may be more structured and standardized, utilizing the same questions in the same manner for every interview. These questions are generally closed-ended. On the other hand, an in-depth unstructured and semistructured interview will utilize open-ended questions, but in a relatively structured sequence. The questions are designed to offer spontaneous responses and open the opportunity for more in-depth follow-up. See table 2.2 for examples.

Other considerations in the interview process may include keeping interviews as standardized as feasible, avoiding interpreting for the client, and allowing the client time to respond. In addition, the interview environment should remain as consistent as feasible and distraction free. A safe, confidential environment will help the client respond in a more open and honest manner.

The key to interviewing is to develop the skills for active listening. Active listening is not a new concept but represents time-tested skills for interviewing and interpersonal communications. These skills include nonverbal and verbal aspects of active listening. All of the skills and techniques require that the interviewer be cognizant of the cultural orientation of the recipient and that the therapist practice approaches that are culturally appropriate. Active listening requires the use of multiple techniques that are client centered. Jacobs (2016) offers the following general principles that reflect the active listening skills and techniques used in client interactions and assessment processes.

Nonverbal Aspects of Active Listening in the Assessment Process

Nonverbal active listening includes body language, eye contact, space, and time. Each element of body language needs to be considered in the assessment and interviewing process.

People do interpret the body language of others. It is important for the therapist to portray body language that is receptive and demonstrates interest. Examples may include not crossing your arms but holding them in a relaxed manner with your hands in your lap.

TABLE 2.2 Closed- and Open-Ended Questions

Open-ended questions	Closed-ended questions
What do you perceive as your greatest challenge? What does your daily activity routine look like? Tell me about your friendships and other relationships.	Do you experience challenges on a regular basis? Do you engage in activity on a daily basis? Do you have friends you interact with?

The simple placement of one's arms project a more responsive listener. Try to be as relaxed as possible and avoid fidgeting behavior (e.g., clicking a pen, tapping your foot). Maintaining a relaxed posture releases tensions in the interviewing process.

Eye contact communicates interest and respect. It is not a staring contest but a casual reflection of interest in the person and what they have to say. It is important, however, to educate yourself about the use of eye contact with different cultures, because some perceive eye contact as disrespectful or threatening.

Space includes three subcomponents: position, orientation, and distance (Jacobs, 2016). Each subcomponent reflects different aspects of active listening.

In *positioning*, you may try to match the position of the person with whom you're speaking. If they are sitting, sit; if the person is standing, you may consider standing with them. As a therapist, you need to take the most appropriate approach and position for the individual and situation. Try to find the position that is comfortable and reflects your attention and interest.

Body orientation refers to how the therapist turns their body in relation to the consumer. Generally, the therapist would face the individual they are interviewing. The therapist needs to be aware of the cultural background of the client with whom they are communicating, because the body orientation of the therapist will need to accommodate the interviewee. As pointed out by Jacobs (2016), some cultures find it offensive for the person to allow the soles of their shoes to be seen. It is essential for the therapist to be aware of the interpretation of orientation by different cultures.

Distance is the space between those communicating. Different cultures utilize varying practices on personal space. Be aware of the culture and the concept of personal space in the interview process.

Time refers to being aware of the needs of the individual regarding the amount of time and attention needed for the interview process. While service delivery in today's health care arena emphasizes efficiency, taking sufficient time in the interviewing and assessment process is critical in producing effective outcomes.

Verbal Aspects of Active Listening in the Assessment Process

As with nonverbal aspects of active listening, there are also verbal aspects to active listening in the interview process. These include voice tone and the use of probing questions, attentive silence, restating and reflecting, and synthesizing (Brédart et al., 2014).

Voice tone aids in keeping the interview nonthreatening. According to Jacobs (2016), "a pleasant tone of voice and choosing soothing words" are one of the keys to the verbal aspects of active listening and will aid in the assessment process by helping the client feel more relaxed and less threatened. Jacobs goes on to indicate that a lower tone of voice is more soothing than a high, shrill pitch. Included in tone and verbal communication are affirmative "uh-huh" and "hmm" with a physical nod of the head to emphasize understanding and attentiveness.

Attentive silence is another technique that may assist in the interview process. This is not a deafening silence, but a reasonable pause. The attentive silence allows the therapist and the client time to reflect. Often, the client will expound on the question to keep the discussion moving, allowing more information for the therapist to consider.

Student Exercise in Nonverbal Active Listening

Using your smart phone or other means of recording, record mock interviews with one of your peers. The interview can be about family background or interests or school. Play back the recording and make notes of your own nonverbal behaviors during the interview.

Another effective verbal technique is restating and reflecting. In restating and reflecting, the therapist will restate in their own words (not the same words of the client) their understanding of the response. Reflecting back allows the client an opportunity to continue or further clarify a response.

Finally, synthesizing will assist the therapist in summarizing key aspects of the interview. Synthesizing also allows the client an opportunity to clarify any misunderstanding. It also shows the client that you were attentive to their concerns in the interview process (Brédart et al., 2014).

Observation as an Aspect of Client Assessment

Essential to client assessment is consumer observation. Often, the recreational therapist must use observation of the client's behavior or functional performance while on the unit or while engaged in a specifically designed treatment activity. Assessment tools such as the Functional Independence Measure (FIM) and the ICF use observation as a key element in assessing functional performance. The ICF was developed in order to optimize on a common language across clinicians and settings (WHO, 2001). In utilizing observation, however, there are key activities that should be employed to ensure that an observation is both valid and reliable.

1. Specify or define what you are observing. It is important for the therapist to determine exactly what behaviors are of interest and what those behaviors look like. The behavior or functional skill should look the same across coworkers (interrater reliability).

2. Train all personnel on the observation instrument and how to discriminate on the functional area being observed.

3. Periodically check for interrater reliability to ensure consistency of observation, because consumer assessment is a dynamic process.

4. Use a standardized environment during the assessment process. As noted in the ICF,

   To assess the full ability of the individual, one would need to have a 'standardized' environment to neutralize the varying impact of different environments on the ability of the individual. This standardized environment may be: (a) an actual environment commonly used for capacity assessment in test settings; or (b) in cases where this is not possible, an assumed environment which can be thought to have a uniform impact. (WHO, 2001, p. 15)

Observation in the assessment process is essential, particularly when applying coding mechanisms like the ICF or FIM. It is essential that everyone engaged in the assessment process is indeed speaking the same language and rating observations consistently.

Summary

While it is not likely to find an instrument that will address all of the needs of your consumer, identifying the specific functional areas you will be addressing as a therapist can help identify a sound instrument and focus your treatment outcomes. In summary, key areas to consider in the assessment process will include the following:

- Focus on your consumers' dominant needs. In health care, RT professionals cannot do everything and should focus on the most critical health and functional outcome needs of their consumer within their scope of practice and the mission of the agency they represent.

- Identify what variables or areas of functioning you will be addressing. Your areas of functional concern will be driven by consumer need and your own competencies.

- Ensure that each recreational therapist and RT assistant working under the supervision of the therapist is trained in administering the instrument and process.

- Ensure consistency in assessment processes and procedures, carefully reviewing assessment results for inconsistencies and periodically reviewing the process.
- Locate potential assessment instruments and ensure, through the literature, that the instruments are valid, reliable, and practical for use with your consumer.

Ultimately, the recreational therapist should be using the results of the assessment process to determine treatment plans and to focus treatment on the documented needs of the consumer. As practicing recreational therapists, there will be an ongoing need to continually keep abreast of the literature as it relates to assessment, including attending conferences that focus on functional outcome strategies and assessment competencies. In practice, take time to evolve your service to include sound assessment processes and procedures. The assessment processes will include information from a variety of sources: medical history review, consultation with other health care team members, interviews with the client or family, observations, and a valid and reliable assessment tool that relates to the person's functional needs. If the recreational therapist strives to adhere to the principles of quality assessment practices, the measure of the treatment outcomes will be more tailored to the needs of the consumer, more discrete in focus, and more meaningful for the consumers served.

REFLECTION QUESTIONS

1. What does it mean for an assessment instrument to be valid?
2. To what does *instrument reliability* refer?
3. How might a team of recreational therapists ensure that they are consistent in the administration of a client assessment?
4. Give one example of an open-ended question and one example of a closed-ended question.
5. Write a list of behaviors or functional skills you might observe for each of the following and compare lists with a partner for consistency:
   - Undertaking single step tasks
   - Interacting with other people
   - Maintaining static balance
   - Maintaining dynamic balance
   - Communicating effectively with peers

   How does the ICF define these functional areas?

REFERENCES

American Therapeutic Recreation Association. (2013). *Standards for the practice of recreational therapy.* Hattiesburg, MS: Author.

Brédart, A., Marrel, A., Abetz-Webb, L., Lasch, L., & Acquadro, C. (2014). Interviewing to develop patient reported outcome (PRO) measures for clinical research: Eliciting patients' experience. *Health and Quality of Life Outcomes, 12*(15). Retrieved from www.hqlo.com/content/12/1/15

Cook, D.A., & Beckman, T.J. (2006). Current concepts in validity and reliability for psychometric instruments: Theory and application. *The American Journal of Medicine, 119.* Retrieved April 12, 2018, from www.famecourse.org/pdf/CookandBeckman.pdf

Jacobs, G.A. (2016). *Community-based psychological first aid: A practical guide to helping individuals and communities during difficult times.* Portsmouth, NH: Butterworth-Heinemann. Retrieved from https://doi.org/10.1016/B978-0-12-804292-2.00006-5

McLeod, S.A. (2013). What is validity? Retrieved from www.simplypsychology.org/validity.html

Podsiadlo, D., & Richardson, S. (1991, Feb.). The timed "up & go": A test of basic functional mobility for frail elderly persons. *Journal of the American Geriatrics Society, 39*(2), 142-148.

Richter, R.R., & Werner, C.M. (2015). Understanding validity in evidence-based medicine. *Evidence Based Medicine, 26*(2), 149-154.

Sullivan, G.M. (2011). A primer on the validity of assessment instruments. *Journal of Graduate Medical Education, 3*(2), 119-120.

Trochim, W., & Web Center for Social Research Methods. (2018). Validity and reliability. Retrieved July 9, 2018, from https://socialresearchmethods.net/kb/relandval.php

World Health Organization. (2001). *International classification of functioning, disability and health.* Geneva, Switzerland: Author.

ADDITIONAL RESOURCES

Ferrari, M., Ahmad, F., Shakya, Y., Ledwos, C., & McKenzie, K. (2016). Computer-assisted client assessment survey for mental health: Patient and health provider perspectives. *BMC Health Services Research, 16*(1). Retrieved from http://link.galegroup.com.jproxy.lib.ecu.edu/apps/doc/A464561077/HRCA?u=ncliveecu&sid=HRCA&xid=effab7eb

McLeod, S.A. (2007). What is reliability? Retrieved from www.simplypsychology.org/reliability.html

Morgan, S. (2015). *Working with strengths: The developmental pathway to addiction recovery.* Pavilion, ProQuest Ebook Central, https://ebookcentral.proquest.com/lib/east-carolina/detail.action?docID=3384819

CHAPTER 3

Understanding the *International Classification for Functioning, Disability and Health* (ICF) and Consumer Assessment

Thomas K. Skalko, PhD, LRT/CTRS, FDRT

LEARNING OBJECTIVES

Upon completion of the text, the student will demonstrate:

- Knowledge of the World Health Organization's (WHO) *International Classification of Functioning, Disability and Health* (ICF) as a method of assessing individual functioning and the impact of activity limitations and restrictions to participation in life activities, independence, satisfaction, and quality of life.

- Skill in applying ICF functional domains to client assessment.

The promotion of full engagement in the life of the community for persons with varying levels of functioning is the ultimate goal of all health care and social service professionals. This goal is accomplished through effective assessment, treatment to improve functional capacity, community-based programs and services, and policies and practices that facilitate community participation and inclusion. This chapter is designed to offer an introduction to the *International Classification of Functioning, Disability and Health* (ICF) and to explore assessment as it relates the application of the ICF in addressing functioning and the community engagement of all citizens.

On May 22, 2001, through resolution WHA 54.21, all 191 members of the World Health Organization's member states endorsed the *International Classification of Functioning, Disability and Health* (ICF) model as a framework for classifying and understanding disability and health (WHO, 2017). Prior to the introduction of the ICF, the *International Statistical Classification of Disease and Related Health Problems* (ICD) was used to provide an etiological framework to classify diagnosis, disorder, disease, and other health conditions (i.e., medical model) (Stucki, 2012). The endorsement of the ICF provided a shift in how health care and human service professionals address health and disability globally (biopsychosocial model). By using the current ICD-11 in conjunction with the ICF, providers are able to gain a more complete understanding of the individual, their condition, and the impacts of a disability, disease, or disorder on functioning (WHO, 2001, 2002).

"The *International Classification of Functioning, Disability and Health*, known more commonly as ICF, provides a standard language and framework for the description of health and health-related states" (WHO, 2002, p. 2). The ICF serves as a universal biopsychosocial model for measuring and classifying human functioning, including disability and health. In summary, the ICF "is the conceptual basis for the definition, measurement and policy formulations for health and disability" (WHO, 2002, p. 2). The ICF is "not only about people with disabilities; it is about *all people*" (WHO, 2001, p. 7). The ICF shifts the perspective from a focus on disability to an emphasis on an individual's overall level of health and functioning, including the technology, environment, and policies that affect their overall health. After all, "functioning is what matters to the health professional's patients" (Bickenbach, 2012, p. 3).

This paradigm shift in understanding and classifying functioning (as opposed to disability, condition, or disease) in a standard environment allows service providers and policy makers to explore how the assessed functioning of the individual affects their health and engagement in the life of the community. Nearly all persons possess some impairment in body structure, body function, or activity and participation in life. Therefore, it is essential for health and human service providers to understand how an individual's functioning affects their engagement in life and what strategies can be used to minimize their impairment, whether through intervention strategies, environmental modifications, or policy changes. The initial step in this process is the functional assessment of the individual, which may include access to technologies, economic supports, environmental modifications, or legislative policy.

Understanding the ICF Model

To apply the coding of the ICF for effective service delivery, one needs to first understand how to utilize the ICF as a means to classify the full functioning of the individual, perhaps beginning with a diagnosis from the ICD-11 (see www.who.int/classifications/icd/revision/icdprojectplan2015to2018.pdf?ua=1). The ICD-11 is a medical coding system for documenting diagnoses, signs of illness, symptoms of a condition, and social circumstances. Unlike the ICF, which focuses on functioning, the ICD offers some insights into the etiological classification by diagnosis of health condition, disorder, or disease. Coupled with the ICF, both classification schemes offer a relatively full picture of the medical and biopsychosocial aspects of the individual (Stucki, 2012).

Because this chapter focuses on understanding the ICF and demonstrating its connection to assessment, a full understanding of the ICF is of value to the reader. The ICF is a hierarchical structure consisting of two parts, each with two components. Part 1, functioning and disability, is broken into the components (1) body functions and structures, and (2) activities and participation. Part 2, contextual factors, is broken into (1) environmental factors and (2) personal factors. (Note: Types of personal factors are identified for clarity but are not classified, because every person has unique personal factors and the classification of every person's personal factors would be impossible.) In the ICF, "Each component (except personal factors) can be expressed in both positive and negative terms" (WHO, 2001, p. 10).

The ICF

domains are classified from body, individual and societal perspectives by means of two lists: a list of body functions and structure, and a list of domains of activity and participation. In the ICF, the term functioning refers to all body functions, activities and participation. The term disability is similarly an umbrella term for impairments, activity limitations and participation restrictions. The ICF also lists environmental factors that interact with all these components. (WHO, 2002, p. 2)

The ICF is

a classification of health and health-related domains—domains that help us to describe changes in body function and structure, what a person with a health condition can do in a standard environment (their level of capacity), as well as what they actually do in their usual environment (their level of performance). (WHO, 2002, p. 2)

Let's break down these concepts in order to better understand the ICF. The ICF model, as shown in figure 3.1, offers a coding system that begins with the recognition of a health condition. As delineated in the ICF, a health condition (disorder or disease) generally affects some physical (biological) or functional aspect of the individual's body structure or body function. Changes or impacts on body structure—for example, a spinal cord injury, limb amputation, or even pregnancy or aging—may affect an individual's functioning in multiple domains. The affected body structure or function affects the activities and participation of the individual in the life of the community. In addition, environmental factors contextually affect the individual in a positive (facilitator) or negative (barrier) manner. Remember, since every

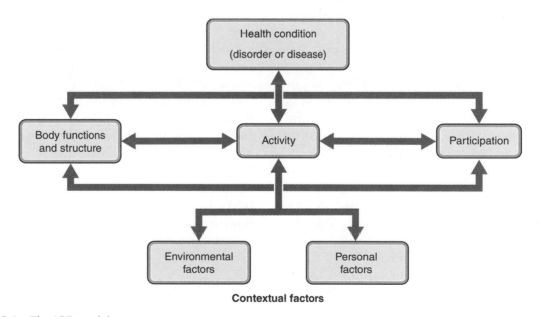

FIGURE 3.1 The ICF model.

Adapted by permission from *International Classification of Functioning, Disability, and Health*, pg. 18, copyright 2001 (Geneva, World Health Organization); Adapted from B. Prodinger et al., "Toward the ICF Rehabilitation Set: A Minimal Generic Set of Domains for Rehabilitation as a Health Strategy," *Archives of Physical Medicine and Rehabilitation* 97, no. 6 (2016): 875-884.

person is unique, the ICF does not include personal factors in the classification system but does provide examples of factors to consider.

The impact on body structure and body function has implications for the ability of the individual to engage in activities (execution of a task) and participation (engagement in the life of the community). It is important to note that the community may range from the broader environment (e.g., city or neighborhood) to home or residential facility.

Unlike what one may perceive from the term *activities* (e.g., a recreational event), activities under the ICF are more discrete. Activities within the ICF refer to the specific execution of a task like manipulating objects (i.e., holding a pencil), focusing attention, or walking on different surfaces. Participation, on the other hand, may include moving around within a facility or using transportation. Together, the concepts of activities and participation are a bit different within the ICF model than how they are often used within recreational therapy practice. In recreational therapy service delivery, we often think of an activity as a game or manual arts project or exercise in a group. In the ICF model, as noted, an activity may be grasping an object, balancing on a foot, or making a decision. If a consumer cannot grasp a paint brush, they will not be able to participate in a painting experience or event. Therefore, participation in a community art class may not be possible unless the therapist assists the consumer in acquiring the skill of grasping or making a modification. So, it is important to note that the ICF classifies the functional performance of the discrete tasks or actions needed to participate in life situations. As therapists, we want to be able to assess one's functioning in such discrete tasks so that we can improve the functioning, design adapted supplies, or modify the activity to enhance engagement (participation).

In addition to body structure, body function, and activities and participation, environmental and personal factors also affect the functioning of the individual. Environmental elements include products and technology, natural environment and human-made changes to the environment, support and relationships, attitudes of others, and services, systems, and policies. The qualities (or lack thereof) of the environment, including technology, affect the ability of an individual to address functioning (e.g., a prosthetic device) and, therefore, engagement in the life of the community (see figure 3.1). Remember that personal factors, such as gender, ethnicity, religious beliefs, cultural morays, and family upbringing, are not coded because every individual is unique.

To understand the model, a brief description of each element is of value. Table 3.1 offers an explanation/definition of each component of the ICF (Rauch, Luckenkemper, & Cieza, 2012; WHO, 2001). Unlike earlier linear models of disability, the ICF model is a dynamic and interactive model that reflects the functioning of the individual and recognizes the impacts of each element in an individual's life. Each component interacts with the other components depicting this dynamic relationship. For instance, when an individual's body structure is changed, there is a subsequent impact on body function, activities, and engagement in the life of the community. When an individual engages in an activity that improves body function or structure, there is a resulting impact on activities that may also affect participation in the community. The ICF is about classifying functioning and includes those environmental factors that can facilitate functioning and engagement or serve as barriers to one's functioning.

The following sections offer a brief explanation of each element of the ICF. It is important to recognize the dynamic relationship between each element and the resulting positive or negative impact on an individual. The health condition has an impact on body structure, body function, activities, participation, and environment functioning, each altering the functioning of the individual.

Health Condition

All humans possess some health conditions that have positive and negative implications for daily functioning. Many times, these health

TABLE 3.1 Definitions of the Components of Model of Functioning and Disability

Positive	Negative
Body functions are physiological functions of body systems (including psychological functions). *Body structures* are anatomical parts of the body such as organs, limbs, and their components. *Activity* is the execution of a task or action by an individual. *Participation* is involvement in a life situation.	*Impairments* are problems in body function or structure such as a significant deviation or loss. *Activity limitations* are difficulties an individual may have in executing activities. *Participation restrictions* are problems an individual may experience in involvement in life situations.
Facilitators	**Barriers**
Environmental factors make up the physical, social, and attitudinal environment in which people live and conduct their lives. *Personal factors* are the particular background of an individual's life and living and comprise features of the individual that are not part of the health condition or health state. (These factors may include gender, race, age, other health conditions, fitness, lifestyle, habits, upbringing, coping styles, social background, education, profession, past and current experiences, etc.)	

From Bickenbach, Cieza, Rauch, & Stucki (2012, p. 6); WHO (2001, p. 10).

conditions result in little or no impairment, but other times they can result in significant functional impairment and disability. The individual's health condition, in turn, has a resulting impact on body structure or body function and activities and participation in the community. Some individuals are born with or acquire a condition during their life span. In addition, the aging process alone may have impacts on tolerance for activity, balance, cognition, and muscular strength, as well as on body structure, leading to muscle atrophy or reduced cardiovascular efficiencies. These conditions affect daily functioning in a host of activities.

Body Structure

The changes in body structure as the result of a health condition also affect an individual's body functioning. Positive and negative impacts on body function affect the individual's participation in activities and engagement in community living. For example, if consumers are provided exercise, tai chi, or yoga in the rehabilitation or community setting, the strategies may improve lower extremity muscular strength and balance and may therefore

positively affect the person's ability to engage in a wider range of activities and tasks for daily life (Gatts & Woollacott, 2007; Ge, 2002; Hakim, Kotroba, Cours, Teel, & Leininger, 2010). There are a wide range of body structure impairments that affect engagement in activities and community living. Improvements in any one factor of body structure has resultant impacts on body function (WHO, 2001).

Body Function

Body function refers to the physiological function of body systems. When body functions are affected by an impairment or other changes in the body (e.g., pregnancy), several aspects of both body structure and body function are affected (e.g., balance, ambulation, tolerance of activity, emotional control). Many of these impacts on body function can be addressed through well-designed interventions or community-based programs, including exercise, support groups, and relaxation and stress management. The key, however, is to be able to assess aspects of body function within the scope of recreational therapy practice (see CAAHEP-CARTE *Standards and Guidelines for Recreational Therapy Accreditation*). Therefore, the utilization of valid and reliable assessment instruments and processes becomes essential. As noted by King (2014), assessment, as a process, includes a diverse set of inputs that support and clarify the assessment outcomes. This set of inputs allows for the application of the ICF in the classification of functioning.

Other impacts on body function, such as mental function (including concentration, orientation, temperament, attention, memory, and anxiety management), joint function, movement function, and cardiovascular and respiratory system function, can all be assessed and addressed through therapeutic interventions and through a range of health care and community-based programs. To illustrate, treatment-based stress management interventions may address anxiety-related conditions; similarly, community-based yoga and other forms of physical activity may also serve as management and prevention approaches to addressing stress (Tennstedt, Howland, Lachman, Peterson, Kasten, & Jette, 1998). The same applies when exercise can be used to improve cardiovascular function and activity tolerance (Cardenas, Henderson, & Wilson, 2009; Erikssen, Liestol, Bjornholt, Thaulow, Sandvik, & Erikssen, 1998; Lees, Clark, Nigg, & Newman, 2005).

Activities and Participation

As noted earlier, unlike what is typically reflected as an activity in recreational therapy practice (e.g., arts and crafts), activities under the ICF are the execution of a specific task or action of the individual. Examples may include the ability to give and receive social cues or to apply knowledge to solve problems. During the assessment process, an individual with an acquired brain injury may have difficulty with social cues in relationships or with solving simple problems. For simple problems, the recreational therapist may utilize a treatment activity to improve the ability to solve simple one, two, or three step problems and then advance to more complex problem solving. Community-based recreational therapy and social service providers may also use problem-solving activities to stimulate cognition in older adults in order to maintain and improve brain function as

a preventative approach to address the impacts of the aging process and to improve functioning for a host of daily tasks (Zettel-Watson, Suen, Wehbe, Rutledge, & Cherry, 2017).

Engagement in the life of the community (participation) is the ultimate outcome for the individual and the goal of all allied health and social service disciplines. Treatment, community service providers, human service policies, and environmental modifications may all affect the individual's engagement. Available services should be designed to enhance inclusion and participation of all citizens. The goal is full engagement and the provision of those services that facilitate the ability of the individual to maintain effective community living and participation (Bickenbach, 2012; WHO, 2001).

Environmental Factors

The "physical, social, and attitudinal environment in which people live and conduct their lives" comprises environmental factors of the ICF (WHO, 2001, p. 10). All allied health and social service professionals concern themselves with issues related to environmental factors. These issues include available technologies, policy formulation, facility and environmental accessibility, economic systems, supportive relationships, and societal attitudes.

In the ICF, environmental factors may be either an asset (facilitator) or a liability (barrier). For instance, a supportive family is considered a facilitator to functioning and community engagement. However, an unsupportive family will negatively affect a person's functioning and, in turn, is considered a barrier to functioning and successful community participation. The same holds true for traditional environmental factors such as accessible facilities, mobility friendly communities, and social security systems (Khumalo, Van Herden, & Skalko, in press).

Within clinical practices, across allied health professions, the therapist (recreational, physical, or occupational) utilizes technologies to promote functioning and community participation. In addition, each discipline contributes to the promotion of accessible facilities, family and peer relationships, and policies that facilitate community inclusion and participation.

In the community setting, recreational therapy and leisure service professionals play an essential role in ensuring that community recreation facilities are accessible and that programs are designed for inclusion. An example would be ensuring that community playgrounds are designed to be accommodating and accessible. Paths, picnic tables, swings, and other forms of play equipment should include options that promote participation of all citizens. Safe and accommodating home environments can be assessed for effective community living. Each environment can be assessed to facilitate use through accommodations. While a challenge for many individuals and communities, accessible facilities using universal design principles should be a priority for all agencies and all health and social service professionals (Centre for Excellence in Universal Design, 2018).

Personal Factors

Like environmental factors, personal factors are considered contextual but are not coded within the ICF. "Personal factors are the particular background of an individual's life and living, and comprise features of the individual that are not part of a health condition or health states" (WHO, 2001, p. 17). Examples include age, race, gender, lifestyle, habits, social and cultural background, past and current life experiences, and individual psychological assets, among other attributes. Each of these may play a role in the functioning of the individual but are too varied to be classified and impossible to rate with regard to impacts, either positive or negative. Despite this, they are included in the model, because personal factors "may have an impact on the outcome of various interventions" (WHO, 2001, p. 17).

ICF Classification and Coding

The classification hierarchy of the ICF begins with a chapter (first level of classification). Each chapter is then further subdivided into basic aspects of the classification called categories and organized by digits into second, third, and fourth levels (Rauch, Luckenkemper, & Cieza, 2012). "Only the Body Function and Body Structure classifications contain fourth-level items" (WHO, 2001, p. 220).

The chapters are coded by the letters s (Body Structure), b (Body Function), d (Activities and Participation), and e (Environmental Factors). Each prefix code (s, b, d, e) is followed by one digit that represents a chapter and three digits for the second level, four for the third level, and five digits for the fourth level. To assist users, the World Health Organization offers an electronic interactive option for the ICF (see http://apps.who.int/classifications/icfbrowser/).

For example, under Body Functions, chapter 7 is (b7), neuromusculoskeletal. As depicted here, the chapter includes functions of movement and mobility and includes functions of joints, bones, reflexes, and muscles.

Functions of the joints and bones (b710-b729)
- b710: Mobility of joint functions
- b715: Stability of joint functions
- b720: Mobility of bone functions

Muscle functions (b730-b749)
- b730: Muscle power functions
- b735: Muscle tone functions
- b740: Muscle endurance functions

Movement functions (b750-b789)
- b750: Motor reflex functions
- b755: Involuntary movement reaction functions
- b760: Control of voluntary movement functions
- b765: Involuntary movement functions
- b770: Gait pattern functions
- b780: Sensations related to muscles and movement functions
- b789, b798, b799: Movement and neuromuscular unspecified/other specified

Let's look more closely one of the areas, b760, control of voluntary movement functions. The area is further classified as follows:

b760: Control of voluntary movement functions

b7600: Control of simple voluntary movements

b7601: Control of complex voluntary movements

b7602: Coordination of voluntary movements

b7603: Supportive functions of the arm or leg (WHO, 2001, p. 100)

Chapter 4 of Activities and Participation is d4, mobility, including changing and maintaining body position (d410-d429). Each category is further "nested" to more exact subcategories. For instance, it includes d410, changing basic body position; d415, maintaining a body position; and d420, transferring oneself.

d410: Changing basic body position

d4100: Lying down

d4101: Squatting

d4102: Kneeling

d4103: Sitting

d4104: Standing

d4105: Bending

d4106: Shifting the body's center of gravity

Under chapter 7, Activities and Participation, Interpersonal Interactions and Relationships (d7), General Interpersonal Interactions, (d710-729), you will find codes including d710 (basic interpersonal interactions) and d720 (complex interpersonal interactions).

d710: Basic interpersonal interactions

d7100: Respect and warmth in relationships

d7101: Appreciation in relationships

d7102: Tolerance in relationships

d7103: Criticism in relationships

d7104: Social cues in relationships

d7105: Physical contact in relationships

So, each area is further classified into more exact subcategories of the area. Recreational therapists often work on knowledge, skills, and abilities for basic interpersonal interactions. The coding, however, does not possess meaning without qualifiers.

Applying Qualifiers

Applying meaning to an ICF code is completed through qualifiers.

The ICF codes require the use of one or more qualifiers, which denote, for example, the magnitude of the level of health or severity of the problem at issue. Qualifiers are coded as one, two, or more numbers after a point. Use of any code should be accompanied by at least one qualifier (WHO, 2001, p. 222).

All of the Part 1 components of the ICF (body function, body structure, and activities and participation) use qualifiers. The first qualifier depicts the magnitude of the level of health or the severity of the problem from full functioning (no problem) to complete disability (complete problem), including intermediate levels of mild, moderate, or severe. In the contextual area of environment, the first qualifier also reflects the extent of problems related to environmental and other supports (barriers), which are denoted with a period (.). Positive influences (facilitators) are denoted with a plus sign (+).

The qualifiers utilize the same generic scale reflecting the problem. The problem may be an impairment, limitation, or barrier depending on the construct. The scale shown in table 3.2 is utilized to reflect levels of functioning, impairment, or barrier/facilitator.

According to the ICF, the broad ranges of percentages allow for standardized assessment to further quantify the impairment, capacity limitations, performance problems, or environmental barriers/facilitators (WHO, 2001). There are, however, coding variations in each category, b, d, s, and e.

Body Function

For Body Function, b7602 (coordination of voluntary movements), the use of b7602.3 indicates a severe impairment in the coordination of voluntary movements. A code of b7602.2 indicates a moderate problem with the coordination of voluntary movements. These ratings would be associated with the results of a complete picture of the individual, including ICD-11 diagnosis, a formal assessment of motor

TABLE 3.2   ICF Rating Scale

xxx.0	No problem/difficulty	None, absent, negligible	0%-4%
xxx.1	Mild problem/difficulty	Slight, low	5%-24%
xxx.2	Moderate problem/difficulty	Medium, fair	25%-49%
xxx.3	Severe problem/difficulty	High, extreme	50%-95%
xxx.4	Complete problem/difficulty	Total	96%-100%
xxx.8	Not specified		
xxx.9	Not applicable		
xxx+0	No facilitator	None, absent, negligible	0%-4%
xxx+1	Mild facilitator	Slight, low	5%-24%
xxx+2	Moderate facilitator	Medium, fair	25%-49%
xxx+3	Substantial facilitator	High, extreme	50%-95%
xxx+4	Complete facilitator	Total	96%-100%
xxx+8	Not specified		
xxx+9	Not applicable		

Adapted by permission from *International Classification of Functioning, Disability and Health*, pg. 179, copyright 2001 (Geneva, World Health Organization).

movement, and observations of the service provider. It is important to note that the Body Function and Body Structure classifications are designed to be parallel so that Chapter 7 in Body Functions (b7) relates to "Neuromus-culoskeletal and movement-related functions" (WHO, 2001, p. 35) and Chapter 7 in Body Structures (s7) covers "Structures related to movement" (p. 38). See table 3.3 for a summary of body functions and structures.

TABLE 3.3   Body Functions and Body Structures

Body function	Body structure
Mental functions (b1)	Structures of the nervous system (s1)
Sensory functions and pain (b2)	The eye, ear and related structures (s2)
Voice and speech functions (b3)	Structures involved in voice and speech (s3)
Functions of the cardiovascular, haematological, immunological, and respiratory systems (b4)	Structures of the cardiovascular, immunological and respiratory systems (s4)
Functions of the digestive, metabolic and endocrine systems (b5)	Structures related to the digestive, metabolic and endocrine systems (s5)
Genitourinary and reproductive functions (b6)	Structures related to the genitourinary and reproductive systems (s6)
Neuromusculoskeletal and movement-related functions (b7)	Structures related to movement (s7)
Functions of the skin and related structures (b8)	Skin and related structures (s8)

WHO (2001).

Body Structure

Body structure refers to "anatomical parts of the body such as organs, limbs, and their components. Impairments are problems in body function or structure as a significant deviation or loss" (WHO, 2001, p. 228). The coding for body structure, however, uses three separate qualifiers. The first qualifier reflects the extent of impairment. The second qualifier indicates the nature of the impairment. The third qualifier addresses the location of impairment.

Table 3.4 reflects the coding for body structure. As an example, the code s7501 is structure of the lower leg. The code s75010.411 would indicate (4) a complete impairment of the bones of the lower leg, (1) total absence, (1) right side. This person has an absence of his lower right leg. The exercises later in this chapter will provide further opportunities to use body structure coding.

Activities and Participation

Activities involve the execution of a task or action, and participation is involvement in a life situation. "*Activity limitations* are difficulties an individual may have in executing activities. *Participation restrictions* are problems an individual may experience in involvement in life situations" (WHO, 2001, p. 229). So, under Activities and Participation, one or both may be coded under the ICF, where an *activity limitation* will reflect the individual's ability to execute a given task or activity and a *participation restriction* will reflect the impact that the activity has on engagement in life activities.

For example, walking (d450) is defined as, "Moving along a surface on foot, step by step, so that one foot is always on the ground, such as when strolling, sauntering, walking forwards, backwards, or sideways " (WHO, 2001, p. 144).

d4500: Walking short distances

d4501: Walking long distances

d4502: Walking on different surfaces

d4503: Walking around obstacles

d4508: Walking, other specified

d4509: Walking, unspecified

(Note that d4508 is used when there is "insufficient information to specify the severity of the impairment"; and d4509 is used "where it is inappropriate to apply a particular code" (WHO, 2001, pp. 226-227).

The code alone, however, has no meaning without the use of qualifiers. In the coding of Activities and Participation, additional qualifying codes may also be applied. "The two qualifiers for the Activities and Participation component are the performance qualifier and the capacity qualifier" (WHO, 2001, p. 123). The code begins with the area of domain followed

TABLE 3.4 Scaling of Qualifiers for Body Structure

First qualifier Extent of impairment	Second qualifier Nature of impairment	Third qualifier Location of impairment
xxx.0: No impairment	0: No change in structure	0: More than one region
xxx.1: Mild impairment	1: Total absence	1: Right
xxx.2: Moderate impairment	2: Partial absence	2: Left
xxx.3: Severe impairment	3: Additional part	3: Both sides
xxx.4: Complete impairment	4: Aberrant dimensions	4: Front
xxx.8: Not specified	5: Discontinuity	5: Back
xxx.9: Not applicable	6: Deviating position	6: Proximal
	7: Qualitative changes in structure, including accumulation of fluid	7: Distal
	8: Not specified	8: Not specified
	9: Not applicable	9: Not applicable

Adapted by permission from *International Classification of Functioning, Disability and Health*, pg. 236, copyright 2001 (Geneva, World Health Organization).

by a period and then a qualifier. The first digit behind the point, following the code, depicts the individual's *performance* in the person's current environment (involvement in a life situation) using the same generic scale of 0 (no problem) to 4 (complete difficulty). The second digit following the individual performance rating is capacity. This digit reflects the individual's capacity without assistance in the area of functioning. This is the highest probable level of functioning a person may reach in the domain at a given moment in time in a standard environment *without* assistance.

So, in the category of walking short distances, the code d4500 would be followed by a period, a rated performance qualifier, and a rated capacity qualifier. The performance qualifier describes what the person does in their current environment (in the context of where they live). The capacity qualifier reflects the projected level of functioning for the individual's ability in that functional category in a uniform environment without assistance or environmental adjustments. In our example of walking a short distance, the environment may be their home or neighborhood and they may be using technological assistance (e.g., a cane or walker). In this example, what would the code d4500.24 reflect? This code indicates that the individual has moderate limitations/difficulties in walking short distances unassisted. In addition, the code indicates that there are complete difficulties in the individual's capacity in walking short distances without the assistance of a cane. As noted in the ICF,

the capacity construct "aims to indicate the highest probable level of functioning that a person may reach in a given domain at a given moment. To assess the full ability of the individual, one would need to have a 'standardized' environment to neutralize the varying impact of different environments on the ability of the individual" (WHO, 2001, p. 229). The assessment of the individual in a standardized environment could be the actual environment used for assessing capacity or an environment that will have a uniform or standard impact on functioning. As with Body Function, the initial codes for Activities and Participation are identical (see table 3.5).

Activities and Participation can also have third- and fourth-level qualifiers, which are optional. The third qualifier indicates capacity with assistance and the fourth reflects performance without assistance. These may be used to offer a more in-depth view of the individual and the potential of intervention strategies. Again, in this example the code d4500.241 would indicate that the individual has moderate difficulty walking short distances (d4500.2). Without assistance (e.g., use of a walking device), the code d4500.24 would reflect a complete difficulty. The third qualifier may be applied in our coding to reflect capacity with assistance. With the use of a quad cane and some strengthening exercises, the person may receive a code of d4500.241, indicating that the individual will have mild difficulty walking short distances. Finally, a code of d4500.2414 would indicate that the individual has a moderate

TABLE 3.5   ICF Rating Scale

xxx.0	No problem/difficulty	None, absent, negligible	0%-4%
xxx.1	Mild problem/difficulty	Slight, low	5%-24%
xxx.2	Moderate problem/difficulty	Medium, fair	25%-49%
xxx.3	Severe problem/difficulty	High, extreme	50%-95%
xxx.4	Complete problem/difficulty	Total	96%-100%
xxx.8	Not specified		
xxx.9	Not applicable		

Reprinted by permission from *International Classification of Functioning, Disability and Health*, pg. 230, copyright 2001 (Geneva, World Health Organization).

difficulty walking short distances (performance) (d4500.2); that the activity would be a complete impairment without assistance (d4500.24); and that the person's capacity with assistance (use of a cane) and some designed exercises would only demonstrate mild difficulty (d4500.241). Without that assistance, the person would have complete difficulty in executing the activity (walking short distances) (d4500.2414).

It is important to note that the typical classification only qualifies performance and capacity. The extended classification qualifiers are not generally utilized except when clinically needed.

Environmental Factors

When coding environmental factors, the physical, social, and attitudinal environment in which the individual will conduct their life must be assessed. Environmental factors can be coded alone without relating to the coding of body function, body structure, or activities and participation. Environmental factors, however, can also be coded separately for every component. Finally, environmental factors can be coded for activities and participation in every item (WHO, 2001).

Coding for environmental factors uses the same scale as the body function and activities and participation, but with a variation. As reflected in table 3.6, environmental factors are coded as to whether the factor is a facilitator or a barrier.

It is important to note that environmental factors be considered in relation to accessibility, consistency and dependability of resources, and how frequently the person experiences the facilitator or barrier. In coding, a barrier receives a period (.) followed by the scale. For facilitators, a plus sign (+) is used, without the period, followed by the scale digit. So using the ICF, what would the code e1650+4 indicate? (Answer: Financial assets are a complete facilitator.) What would the code e1650.3 reflect? (Answer: Financial assets are a severe barrier). For a compilation of all four factors, see table 3.7.

TABLE 3.6   Coding for Environmental Factors

Barrier	Facilitator
xxx.0: No barrier	xxx+0: No facilitator
xxx.1: Mild barrier	xxx+1: Mild facilitator
xxx.2: Moderate barrier	xxx+2: Moderate facilitator
xxx.3: Severe barrier	xxx+3: Substantial facilitator
xxx.4: Complete barrier	xxx+4: Complete facilitator
xxx.8: Not specified	xxx+8: Not specified
xxx.9: Not applicable	xxx+9: Not applicable

Adapted by permission from *International Classification of Functioning, Disability and Health*, pg. 247, copyright 2001 (Geneva, World Health Organization).

TABLE 3.7   Compilation of Qualifiers for the ICF

Component	First qualifier	Second qualifier	Third qualifier
Body functions	Extent of impairment		
	0: No impairment 1: Mild impairment 2: Moderate impairment 3: Severe impairment 4: Complete impairment 8: Not specified 9: Not applicable		

Component	First qualifier	Second qualifier	Third qualifier
Body structure	Extent of impairment	Nature of impairment	Location of impairment
	0: No impairment 1: Mild impairment 2: Moderate impairment 3: Severe impairment 4: Complete impairment 8: Not specified 9: Not applicable	0: No change in structure 1: Total absence 2: Partial absence 3: Additional part 4: Aberrant dimension 5: Discontinuity 6: Deviating position 7: Qualitative changes in structure, including accumulation of fluid 8: Not specified 9: Not applicable	0: More than one region 1: Right 2: Left 3: Both sides 4: Front 5: Back 6: Proximal 7: Distal 8: Not specified 9: Not applicable
Activities and participation	Extent of difficulty in performance in current environment	Extent of difficulty in capacity to execute a task or action	
	0: No difficulty 1: Mild difficulty 2: Moderate difficulty 3: Severe difficulty 4: Complete difficulty 8: Not specified 9: Not applicable	0: No difficulty 1: Mild difficulty 2: Moderate difficulty 3: Severe difficulty 4: Complete difficulty 8: Not specified 9: Not applicable	
Environmental factors	Extent of impact of factors in the environment		
	0: No barrier 1: Mild barrier 2: Moderate barrier 3: Severe barrier 4: Complete barrier 8: Not specified 9: Not applicable +0: No facilitator +1: Mild facilitator +2: Moderate facilitator +3: Substantial facilitator +4: Complete facilitator +8: Not specified +9: Not applicable		

Adapted by permission from *International Classification of Functioning, Disability and Health*, pg. 242, copyright 2001 (Geneva, World Health Organization), as presented by Rauch, Luckenkemper & Cieza, 2012.

CODING EXERCISE
Coding Examples to Test Your Understanding

Determine the ICF codes for the following individuals.

Robert: Robert is a 37-year-old male. Robert currently demonstrates a severe impairment in regulating his emotions. Robert has been diagnosed with an anxiety disorder. Observation and a formal assessment indicate that Robert has severe difficulty handling stressful situations. What would be Robert's ICF codes for both body functioning and activities and participation?

Based on the clinical treatment planning process, it was determined that if the agency does not do anything, Robert will continue to have severe impairment in regulating his emotions and handling stress. However, enrolling Robert in a formal stress management training program would assist Robert in reducing his stress to a mild level. What is the full ICF code for Robert?

Jennifer: Jennifer is a 68-year-old female with mobility difficulties due to the long-term effects of osteoarthritis (OA) in both knee joints. More specifically, Jennifer's OA has resulted in moderate impairment in both knees due to structural changes. In addition, Jennifer has moderate impairment of muscle strength and endurance in the lower half of her body. With the use of a cane (performance in her environment), she has moderate difficulty walking on uneven surfaces. Jennifer's ability to walk on uneven surfaces is completely difficult without the use of her cane (capacity without assistance). Therapeutically designed exercise should increase muscular strength and result in mild difficulty when walking on uneven surfaces with the aid of her cane. Without intervention, Jennifer will have complete impairment when walking on uneven surfaces. What would be all of Jennifer's ICF codes in this case study?

James: James is in a moderate stage of Alzheimer's disease and will be participating in recreational therapy programs. His symptoms include moderate short-term memory loss, mild problems with orientation to time, and severe difficulties with paying attention. With some structure, James can temporarily improve his attention to topics and tasks to a moderate difficulty code. What would be the ICF codes for James? What programs would you consider to address James' functional capacity?

Angela: Angela is a 25-year-old female injured in an automobile accident. She is referred for RT services. A review of her medical chart contains the following ICF codes about her health condition. Using these codes, classify her body structure and level of functioning for each code. What might the recreational therapist do to assist in her rehabilitation?

s75018.411

b1801.2

b1521.3

b1301.2

d2401.321

d450.441

d9201.441

e1151+3

e1401+3

e310+4

e330.2

Core Sets in the ICF

As noted, the ICF is a comprehensive compilation of codes describing body function, body structure, activities and participation, and environment. Due to the depth and breadth of the coding system, it is impractical to address every person's complete code. As noted by Stucki (2012, p. vii), "Yet, by constructing an exhaustive classification, it was clear that the ICF was not directly usable as a practical tool since, in daily practice, clinicians need only a fraction of the categories found in the ICF." In turn, WHO has developed the ICF Core Sets. The ICF Core Sets serve as practical and invaluable tools for specific health care areas.

Recognizing the complexities and exhaustive classification of the ICF, the Core Sets were developed for health care context to address acute, post-acute, and long-term health conditions and condition groups (Ptyushkin, Selb, & Cieza, 2012). The ICF Core Sets for acute health care context are intended for "the period of time immediately following an injury or onset of a health condition and preceding the early post-acute context" (Rauch et al., 2012, p. 17). Post-acute health care context includes any setting providing services following the acute event. These settings may include the hospital, the rehabilitation facility, or the ambulatory care setting. The long-term health care context includes any setting utilized to address chronic health conditions (Rauch et al., 2012).

In the ICF Core Sets, there are three types of Core Sets: Comprehensive, Brief, and Generic (figure 3.2). Comprehensive ICF Core Sets address the entire array of issues a person in a given setting will experience. The Brief ICF

ICF Rehabilitation Set

9 categories from Body Functions		21 categories from Activities and Participation	
b130	Energy and drive functions (G)	d230	Carrying out daily routine (G)
b134	Sleep functions	d240	Handling stress and other psychological demands
b152	Emotional functions (G)	d410	Changing basic body position
b280	Sensation of pain (G)	d415	Maintaining a body position
b455	Exercise tolerance functions	d420	Transferring oneself
b620	Urination functions	d450	Walking (G)
b640	Sexual functions	d455	Moving around (G)
b710	Mobility of joint functions	d465	Moving around using equipment
b730	Muscle power functions	d470	Using transportation
		d510	Washing oneself
		d520	Caring for body parts
		d530	Toileting
		d540	Dressing
		d550	Eating
		d570	Looking after one's health
		d640	Doing housework
		d660	Assisting others
		d710	Basic interpersonal interactions
		d770	Intimate relationships
		d850	Remunerative employment (G)
		d920	Recreation and leisure

(G) = Categories of the ICF Generic Set

Minimal Set of Environmental Factors

↓

Can be used to complement the ICF Generic and Rehabilitation Sets

FIGURE 3.2 Example of the ICF Rehabilitation Core Set.

Adapted with permission from *ICF Core Sets: Manual for Clinical Practice* by Jerome Bickenbach, Alaros Cieza, Alexandra Rauch, Gerold Stucki, ISBN 978-2-88937-431-7. ©2012 Hogrefe Publishing www.hogrefe.com.

Core Set, taken from the Comprehensive ICF Core Set, addresses dominant problem areas that should be considered for a given health care condition or in a given health care context. The Generic Core Set, which "was developed from a psychometric study" (Ptyushkin et al., 2012, p. 20), can be used to compare a broad range of conditions, settings, and functional areas across countries. It provides an initial, baseline understanding of the individual's functioning. Ultimately, the ICF Core Sets are interdisciplinary in nature and offer a comprehensive assessment of key functional areas across settings and conditions.

As can be noted in figure 3.2, there are multiple areas in which the recreational therapist may classify functioning and treat the individual to improve functional limitations. The Rehabilitation Core Set includes areas such as handling stress. In the rehabilitation setting, the recreational therapist may employ formal stress management interventions to address the functional area. Other areas of concern for the recreational therapist may include assisting the physical therapist in the area of movement by including yoga or tai chi or basic interpersonal interactions through social skills training and social activities.

The ICF Core Sets significantly simplify the daunting nature of the full ICF classification system and promote interdisciplinary assessment and the delivery of interdisciplinary treatment strategies. The above example exemplifies how the ICF promotes interdisciplinary interactions and health care team service delivery. The recreational therapist is working collaboratively with the physical therapist in promoting the full functioning of the individual via RT modalities.

To assist the application of both the Comprehensive and the Brief Core sets, WHO has developed multiple forms to assist the interdisciplinary process. Many of these core set form examples can be found in the *ICF Core Sets: Manual for Clinical Practice* (Bickenbach et al., 2012).

Connecting the ICF and the Assessment and Treatment Planning Process

The ICF is a comprehensive tool to assist clinical decision making in order to provide the most complete functional profile of an individual. The ICF also assists in targeting specific domains for further assessment and performance tracking. In addition, the utilization of the ICF allows for common language across health care providers to focus energies and intervention strategies on functional improvement. Those intervention strategies may range from social and legislative policy change, technology, and strategies for including families and other social supports, to specific strategies to improve body function, body structure, or activities and participation.

For the therapist, the ICF allows a more focused approach to address functional limitations and strategies for collaboration across disciplines. When disciplines can collectively target functional outcomes, the consumer is better served. The ICF also permits the identification of functional areas that require further assessment in order to effectively serve the individual.

Summary

If we embrace the premise that all citizens deserve the right to engage in the life of their community, the ICF model serves as a framework for understanding and classifying functioning and those variables that affect community participation. It is important to remember that the ICF is not disability specific. All persons have some aspect of body structure, body function, activities and participation, and environmental consideration that affects this engagement. Children, older adults, persons in need of visual assistance (e.g., glasses), and persons with disabling conditions can all be classified using the ICF. The model offers a means to classify areas that may require functional intervention strategies, technologies, environmental adjustments, or policy change to promote inclusion.

The Comprehensive Recreational Therapy Service Delivery (CRTSD) model and the ICF are interactive. The CRTSD provides insights on assessment as a process that has a variety of inputs, including comprehensive program planning (CPP), specific program planning (SPP), rapport building, activity and task analysis, and tools for assessment. The ICF provides a systematic process of understanding how personal factors, environmental factors, body function and structure, and health conditions influence activity and participation. The recreational therapist should use the ICF coding or the ICF Core Sets during their assessment process so they can plan and implement their interventions using multiple sources of information in a systematic manner within the ICF. This would then provide a consistent evaluation framework for outcomes measures for the people receiving recreational therapy services and promote the use of a common language among interdisciplinary teams serving persons with disabling conditions. It is the person's functional abilities that drive the treatment strategies and the interdisciplinary process.

REFLECTION QUESTIONS

1. What are the advantages to the recreational therapist in using the ICF in consumer assessment?
2. How can the allied health professional pair the assessment process with the ICF?
3. How can the profession better integrate the ICF into assessment practice and interdisciplinary service delivery?

REFERENCES

Bickenbach, J. (2012). What is functioning and why is it important? In J. Bickenbach, A. Cieza, A. Rauch, & G. Stucki (Eds.), *ICF core sets: Manual for clinical practice* (p. 13). Cambridge, MA: Hogrefe Publishing.

Bickenbach, J., Cieza, A., Rauch, A., & Stucki, G. (Eds). (2012). *ICF core sets: Manual for clinical practice.* Cambridge, MA: Hogrefe Publishing.

Cardenas, D., Henderson, K.A., & Wilson, B.E. (2009). Physical activity and senior games participation: Benefits, constraints, and behaviors. *Journal of Aging & Physical Activity, 17*(2), 135-153. Retrieved from http://search.ebscohost.com.jproxy.lib.ecu.edu/login.aspx?direct=true&db=s3h&AN=37148063&site=ehost-live

Centre for Excellence in Universal Design. (2018). What is universal design. National Disability Authority. Retrieved June 28, 2018, from http://universaldesign.ie/What-is-Universal-Design/

Erikssen, G., Liestol, K., Bjornholt, J., Thaulow, E., Sandvik, L., & Erikssen, J. (1998). Changes in physical fitness and changes in mortality. *The Lancet, 352,* 759-762.

Gatts, S.K., & Woollacott, M. (2007). How tai chi improves balance: Biomechanics of recovery to a walking slip in impaired seniors. *Gait & Posture, 25*(2), 205-214.

Ge, W. (2002). Evaluation of the effectiveness of tai chi for improving balance and preventing falls in the older population—a review [Abstract]. *Journal of the American Geriatric Society, 50*(4), 746-754. doi:10.1046/j.1532-5415.2002.50173.x

Hakim, R.M., Kotroba, E.E., Cours, J.J., Teel, S.S., & Leininger, P.M. (2010). A cross-sectional study of balance-related measures with older adults who participated in tai chi, yoga, or no exercise. *Physical & Occupational Therapy in Geriatrics, 28*(1), 63-74.

Khumalo, B., Van Herden, J., & Skalko, T.K. (in press). State and status of wheelchair basketball facilities in Zimbabwe. In T. Chataika (Ed.), *The Rutledge handbook for disability in South Africa* (pp. 278-289). New York: Routledge.

King, A.D. (2014). *The pick of the litter: Understanding standardized assessment tools and the assessment process with older adults in therapeutic recreation practitioners* (Master's thesis). Dalhousie University, Halifax.

Lees, F.D., Clark, P.G., Nigg, C.R., & Newman, P. (2005). Barriers to exercise behavior among older adults: A focus-group study. *Journal of Aging & Physical Activity, 13*(1), 23. Retrieved from http://search.ebscohost.com/login.aspx?direct=true&db=s3h&AN=15367822&site=e-host-live

Ptyushkin, P., Selb, M., & Cieza, A. (2012). ICF core sets. In J. Bickenbach, A. Cieza, A. Rauch, & G. Stucki (Eds.), *ICF core sets: Manual for clinical practice* (pp. 14-21). Cambridge, MA: Hogrefe Publishing.

Rauch, A., Luckenkemper, M., & Cieza, A. (2012). Introduction to the *International Classification of Functioning, Disability and Health*. In J. Bickenbach, A. Cieza, A. Rauch, & G. Stucki (Eds.), *ICF core sets: Manual for clinical practice* (pp. 4-13). Cambridge, MA: Hogrefe Publishing.

Stucki, G. (2012). Preface. In J. Bickenbach, A. Cieza, A. Rauch, & G. Stucki (Eds.), *ICF core sets: Manual for clinical practice* (pp. vii-viii). Cambridge, MA: Hogrefe Publishing.

Tennstedt, S., Howland, J., Lachman, M., Peterson, E., Kasten, L., & Jette, A. (1998). A randomized, controlled trial of a group intervention to reduce fear of falling and associated activity restriction in older adults [Abstract]. *The Journals of Gerontology, 53*(6), 384-392. Retrieved from www.ncbi.nlm.nih.gov/pubmed/9826971

World Health Organization. (2001). *International classification of functioning, disability and health*. Geneva: Author.

World Health Organization. (2002). *Towards a common language for functioning, disability and health: ICF*. Geneva: Author.

World Health Organization. (2017). *International classification of functioning, disability and health (ICF)*. Retrieved June 1, 2017, from http://www.who.int/classifications/icf/en/

Zettel-Watson, L., Suen, M., Wehbe, L., Rutledge, D.N., & Cherry, B.J. (2017). Aging well: Processing speed inhibition and working memory related to balance and aerobic endurance. *Geriatrics & Gerontology International, 17*(1), 108-115.

ADDITIONAL RESOURCES

Porter, H. (2015). *Recreational therapy for specific diagnoses and conditions*. Enumclaw, WA: Idyll Arbor.

CHAPTER 4

Documentation of Health Outcomes in Recreational Therapy

David P. Loy, PhD, LRT/CTRS

Thomas K. Skalko, PhD, LRT/CTRS, FDRT

LEARNING OBJECTIVES

Upon completion of the text, the student will demonstrate:

- Knowledge of the nature and function of documentation procedures related to assessment and treatment planning.
- Knowledge of different documentation systems and the advantages and disadvantages of each system in recreational therapy.
- Knowledge of medical terminology and abbreviations commonly used in health care charts and documentation.
- Knowledge of best practices for effective documentation in recreational therapy.
- Knowledge of electronic medical records (EMR) and procedures related to digital documentation in recreational therapy.
- Knowledge of future trends and practice directions for documentation in recreational therapy.

For decades, there have been numerous sayings about documentation, but perhaps the most apt is, "If it wasn't written, it didn't happen." The act of documentation across the Assess, Plan, Implement, and Evaluate (APIE) process is essential in health care delivery. The therapist is obligated by regulatory standards and by the *Standards for the Practice of Recreational Therapy* (ATRA, 2013) to document each step of the APIE process. Therefore, the need for the therapist to document each phase of the APIE process is paramount to compliant treatment practices.

In fact, the interpretative guidelines for the Centers for Medicare and Medicaid Services (CMS) *State Operations Manual for Psychiatric Hospitals—Interpretive Guidelines and Survey Procedures (Rev. 149, 10-09-15) Transmittals for Appendix AA Part I—Investigative Procedures Survey Protocol—Psychiatric Hospitals* (2015) address what CMS will look for when evaluating a hospital's compliance with the regulations.

> *Review each patient's record in your sample for compliance with the Special Medical Record Condition's Standards. . . . The primary purpose is to determine what the hospital has committed itself to do for the patient under that patient's treatment plan, whether the treatment plan is being implemented, and whether patients are experiencing the outcomes desired from the treatment plan. (p. 6)*

Therefore, the Centers for Medicare and Medicaid Services (CMS) regulations require the treatment team, including the recreational therapist (RT), to document the patient's treatment process. When auditing assessment outcomes, the CMS utilizes the patient's chart to review the patient's assessment (A) outcomes, the needs of the patient based on the assessment information, the treatment plan (P), including specific treatment outcomes, a review of what services were implemented (I) to address the patient's stated treatment goals, and an evaluation (E) of the patient's progress toward meeting those goals and any modifications to address the patient's progress.

Documentation and the Treatment Planning Process (APIE)

The purpose of documentation is to paint a narrative of the patient's assessed functional limitations and strengths to aid in the establishment of specific, measurable, attainable, realistic, and time-limited (SMART) goals for the patient and outline what the agency will do to meet them (Bexelius, Carlberg, & Lowing, 2018). The documentation of the APIE process allows for the evaluation of the outcomes and treatment services.

The process begins with an assessment of the consumer's functional needs. The assessment will identify the individual's functional limitations and strengths. It is important to remember the complexities of the assessment phase. The assessment should include information from multiple sources and from the use of valid and reliable assessment instruments. It is from this phase of the APIE process that the patient's treatment plan is developed.

From the assessed needs, the therapist and treatment team can establish SMART goals. SMART goals can be linked to one or more chapters of the *International Classification for Functioning, Disability and Health* (ICF), thus addressing specific functional outcomes. In recreational therapy practice, many of the specific outcomes will be included in the Activities and Participation chapter of the ICF. However, other outcomes may be found under Body Function or even Body Structure. The therapist or treatment team can identify those specific functional outcomes to include in the treatment plan.

Once the most applicable outcomes are identified, the goal must be measurable. Focusing on one dimension or area offers a more accurate means to measure the specific outcome. For instance, if the patient's assessment identifies moderate difficulty walking short distances, the ICF classification would be d4500.2. The measure may include: "Following engagement in basic lower body exercises, including walking, the patient will be able to ambulate for 50 feet in 90 seconds."

Now, is the outcome and measure attainable? With daily basic exercise, the ability of walking short distances (50 feet in 90 seconds) may be an attainable outcome. So, thus far, the goal is specific, measurable, and attainable.

By setting time-limited parameters, the goal may read: "Following one week of engagement in basic lower body exercises and walking interventions, the patient will be able to ambulate for 50 feet in 90 seconds."

Thus, the therapist and treatment team have identified a SMART goal for the patient. Utilizing the ICF coding system, the SMART goal will involve different intervention strategies from the members of the interdisciplinary treatment team, with different members focusing on the functional outcome of walking short distances. The physical therapist may engage the individual in lower limb mobility and strengthening, and the recreational therapist may have the individual participate in small group basic exercise and walking at the facility or even in the community.

The use of the ICF to assist in the identification of specific outcomes for the SMART goals helps the entire team in planning interdisciplinary intervention strategies. Each member of the team is working on the same outcomes and using their modalities to respond to the functional needs of the patient.

These outcomes must be documented in the agency's medical records system. Different documentation systems tend to be adopted by agencies to meet the specific treatment needs for the patients served and the agency's record-keeping system; all documentation systems, however, tend to have some basic purposes.

Health Care Monitoring

One purpose of documentation is to provide a system for tracking and communicating outcomes to those practitioners working with an individual. Many health care professionals are responsible for monitoring patients' vital signs, such as body temperature, blood pressure, heart rate, respiration rate, body weight, and appetite (Wilkinson, Treas, & Barnett, 2015).

Because these outcomes are taken at a daily or even hourly rate, documentation tends to be linear to promote tracking of trends over a specific period of time. In addition, these types of documentation systems tend to be "report-at-a-glance" single page flow sheets that allow the practitioner to immediately view the outcomes of the particular patient. Most of the health monitoring information is collected by nursing personnel.

Ongoing Service Delivery

The more relevant documentation for allied health disciplines, including RT, are those systems that track the ongoing treatment service delivery to patients. These systems, whether paper based or electronic, provide structure for the recording of regularly provided treatment notes. Again, the tracking protocol of such treatment notes is adopted by the agency and is mandated on a regular time period appropriate to the care of the clientele and based on regulatory requirements. Because the recreational therapist provides documentation in this format, this chapter will focus on those documentation systems that monitor and provide a record of the ongoing treatment to patients.

Paper-Based Versus Digital Documentation

Another issue related to documentation is the format in which progress notes are provided. For many years, paper-based notes were the only format available for the therapist to document the patient's progress. However, we now live and work in a technological age where digital and online documentation is becoming more prevalent (Charney, 2012). Digital or online documentation is often referred to as *electronic medical records* (EMR) or *electronic health records* (EHR). Because there is an abundance of EMR systems on the market, the specific procedures of using such systems will not be addressed. However, the general use of EMR systems will be discussed later in this chapter. This chapter is written to help the recreational therapist develop effective documentation knowledge and skills that translate to both paper-based and EMR documentation systems.

Best Practices for Effective Documentation

Becoming an effective and efficient medical documenter requires a great deal of time and practice. Some view documentation as more of an art than a skill, because one's style of documentation often changes as a result of professional maturity and even agency-specific protocols and standards. However, there are some very common rules for effective documentation that should be learned and practiced by the recreational therapist.

Write legibly with a black ballpoint pen and only use approved abbreviations. When using paper-based charts, it is recommended the recreational therapist always use a black ballpoint pen to prevent smudges or erasing or altering notes, and to allow others to copy medical charts appropriately. It is also important to only use abbreviations that are approved by the agency. The use of medical abbreviations will be discussed later in this chapter.

Record factual events that can be verified. To be as concise as possible, the recreational therapist should only document vital issues that can be verified. An effective therapist is one with the ability to determine those vital things that should or should not be included in the medical chart. Finally, even if interactions with health care teammates are informative and helpful, the therapist should avoid charting casual conversations with other colleagues. Stick to the facts! The recreational therapist should never document personal feelings or diagnose illnesses that are not verifiable. The use of the word *appears* should be avoided because it often conjures up uncertainty if not substantiated with evidence.

Be concise and specific. The old adage "less is more" certainly applies to the practice of effective documentation. New therapists often have the most difficulty in limiting information within the progress note, attempting to include everything so the note will be effective. However, providing too much information in a progress note is more likely to be ineffective by distracting the reader from the most vital information. It is important for the new therapist to ask, "Is this information vital to painting the narrative picture of the patient's current status? Is it related to the patient's treatment goals?" For example, a therapist entered the following in a progress note: "The patient participated in a game of billiards and lost." A therapist must ask if this information is relevant to the patient's current status. What if the therapist instead wrote "the patient demonstrated improved anger control as he failed to show aggressive emotion after losing a game of billiards"? This entry provides contextual relevance to the patient's anger management and losing the billiards game. The ability to determine what information should be included is a critical skill for the new recreational therapist to learn with experience.

Use descriptive action words. The progress note should provide the reader enough concise information to paint the picture of what transpired. One way to do this is through the use of descriptive action words in medical charts. A descriptive action word is a word or phrase that expresses a participant's physical or mental action. Table 4.1 presents some examples of descriptive action words suitable for medical charting.

Use person-first and enabling terminology. It would be easy for the recreational therapist to include language within progress notes that is limiting to individuals served, particularly when the individuals *are* functionally limited. However, good documentation practice requires the recreational therapist to use language that is both respectful and optimistic of the potential for each individual served. For example, the recreational therapist should always use person-first terminology such as "individual with a spinal cord injury" or "individual with a developmental disability." The language used to describe abilities should be enabling and infer the *potential* of each individual. Therefore, the recreational therapist should never use words such as "afflicted with" or "confined to a wheelchair" when referring to the abilities or deficits of an individual.

Avoid writing in the first person. It is good practice in medical charting for the recreational ther-

TABLE 4.1　Examples of Descriptive Action Words for Documentation

showed	demonstrated	noted
withdrew	offered	resisted
produced	initiated	stated
declined	reported	refused
observed	requested	screamed
attended	finished	verbalized
shifted	required	identified

apist to avoid using first person such as *I* or *me*. Using references to oneself as "the therapist," "CTRS," or "RT student" is more appropriate in progress notes. Similarly, patients or participants should not be referred to by their name or surname. Rather, individuals should be referred to as "patient," "client," or "participant."

Ensure each progress note has accurate identification of the correct patient. In paper-based charting, the therapist may start a note on a blank template. Therefore, it is important to make sure the progress note clearly has the correct patient name (and often patient identification number) so the therapist is sure they are documenting the correct individual. This is particularly the case because personal names are discouraged within note writing. EMR notes often have names and IDs on the note as the therapist accesses it. However, it is good common practice to always be cognizant of the name identified on the note to ensure the correct patient is being documented.

Don't name a second patient. Because the recreational therapist often provides treatment in groups or documents how an individual interacts with others, it may be necessary to reflect upon interaction with others. However, it is important to never refer to other patients in a progress note. Keeping the reference to others

in a generic sense (e.g., "initiated conversation with another patient in group") will prevent the identification of a second patient in the note.

Document occurrences in a timely manner. The accuracy of a medical note is often determined by the therapist's ability to accurately recall things that happened to their patient. Therefore, it is a good practice to document occurrences as soon as they happen, while details are still fresh in the therapist's mind. The longer one waits to document, the more likely key items may be forgotten or inaccurately recalled.

Do not "white out," scratch out, or erase documentation mistakes. Inevitably, errors will be made when making entries in a medical chart. However, it is important for the therapist to correct such errors in a manner that is transparent and allows the reader to see how the mistake was corrected. Scratching out or erasing mistakes may imply to the reader that the therapist is hiding something. Therefore, it is advised to correct a mistake by a) drawing a single line through the incorrect information so as not to prevent reading the incorrect entry, b) insert the correction near the error of the note, and c) initial and date the correction. Figure 4.1 demonstrates how to correct an error in a written note.

FIGURE 4.1　Example of a corrected progress note.

4/24/19 NWB DL

A: The pt. is meeting goals despite being ~~DOB~~ for 2 days. Pt. will benefit from endurance-based interventions next week to regain levels. Pt. remain in ↑ mood + ↑ motivated.---

Corrections in electronic medical records (EMR) are also managed with transparency and should be handled according to the procedures specified in the EMR platform or agency regulations.

Always include signature, credentials, and date. A progress note is not complete until the therapist signs, dates, and provides their credentials. Including these three things indicates who wrote the note, the credentials of the person writing the note, and when the note was written. Whether the individual writing the note has the credential of CTRS, LRT, or RT student, the note should *always* include credentials of the individual writing the entry to signify who is responsible for the note.

Don't amend someone's notes. The therapist is often required to review another therapist's notes when treating an individual with whom they lack familiarity. The recreational therapist may even discover errors in the notes of a colleague. However, the credentialed signature with the note indicates who wrote the note. Correcting another's note, even if innocent, would be fraudulent and unethical. It is the responsibility of the recreational therapist to notify their colleague of the error so that individual can change their note.

Prevent fraud or alteration. When the therapist signs the documentation note, they are indicating that they alone are responsible for the words with the entry. Therefore, it is important for the therapist to prevent fraud or alteration of the notes by others. In a paper-based system, this is done by limiting the amount of available free space, preventing someone from entering information after the note was submitted. Best practices would suggest that the therapist write entirely from left margin to right margin (Quinn & Gordon, 2010). When there is free space at the end of the entry, a single line should be placed from the end of the line to right margin (see figure 4.2).

EMR systems typically have built-in functions that help prevent most fraud and alteration, including password-protected entries; locked notations; audit logs indicating users, dates, and times; and digital error correction protocols. Although not error proof, EMR systems are continuing to help protect the progress note from fraud and alteration (Martinez Monterrubio, Juan, & Raúl, 2015).

Don't record staffing problems, conflicts, incident reports, or words associated with mistakes. The progress note is the official record of treatment for that individual. Progress notes should not include the "dirty laundry" of the agency or therapist. For example, the recreational therapist should never indicate that the patient was not seen because of a "scheduling conflict" or "OT kept patient too long." Similarly, best practices would also suggest that patient incidents or words that imply errors should be placed in other sources of documentation and not the patient notes. Agency administrators and risk managers most likely have separate documentation protocols for incident reports.

Don't document care before it happens. Because documentation is often a very time-consuming task (Clinch & Kellett, 2015), many recreational therapists may be inclined to document routine events before they actually occur. For example, six individuals are committed to attend a community reintegration outing, so the recreational therapist documents each of the six individuals in the chart before the outing departs. Then prior to the outing, one individual becomes ill and is unable to attend. The therapist forgets about the cancellation after the outing and now the progress note inaccurately reflects one individual's participation even though they didn't actually attend. Regardless of the time saved, the recreational therapist should *never* document

---

FIGURE 4.2   Eliminating free space in notes to prevent fraud or alteration.

P: 1) Complete IA c̄ pt., 2) F/U c̄ family to confirm post-D/C resources. 3) Schedule meeting c̄ peer support group to ↑ motivation. -

events before they happen to avoid such documentation oversights.

Effective documentation remains a skill set that grows with practitioner experience. Each therapist develops their own style of documentation, but there are certain common best practices the recreational therapist should utilize to develop their own skill sets. One additional piece of knowledge regarding documentation is knowing the content within effective and efficient progress notes.

Documentation Content: What to Document in the Progress Note

Now that you are familiar with some general rules on documentation, it is important to understand what is included in the body of a progress note. Here are some of the common things documented within the content of the progress note.

Receipt of Referrals or Orders

A physician is responsible for the treatment of patients. Therefore, a physician's order or referral for treatment is made for disciplines to provide treatment. ATRA indicates:

> Many health care facilities have a therapy referral process in place and include RT/TR as part of their standard referral process for other ordered therapies and services. Once the referral for RT is made, usually by the physician or health care professional responsible for the patient's care, an assessment should be completed by the CTRS. On many inpatient program units, a standard order is provided for each new resident "to evaluate for RT/TR services". Patients from outpatient, home health or community programs may also be appropriate for RT, and the referral is done on a case-by-case basis. (ATRA, 2013)

Whether the order or referral for RT service is made as a direct physician's order or a standing order that is provided on admission to the facility, the recreational therapist is responsible for documenting its receipt. This can simply be done by indicating "Physician's orders for RT service received on (date)." The receipt of orders or referral for RT service should always be included in the progress notes to track authority for treatment. Receipt of orders or referral for service within the note is often something examined in an internal or external medical chart audit (ATRA, 2013).

Ongoing Service Delivery

The majority of content within a progress note includes important data related to the treatment goals and progress of the patient served (Burlingame & Blaschko, 2010; Stumbo, 2003; Stumbo & Peterson, 2009). These can often include

- patient's self-report of their health status,
- details of the specific intervention provided (target outcome change addressed, duration),
- changes in patient status,
- complications or adverse reactions that affect treatment,
- factors that change the intervention,
- consistency of behavior or new patterns of behavior,
- progression/regression toward patient goal attainment,
- appropriate/inappropriate communication with other patients, providers of care, or the patient's family,
- follow-through or initiative with established goals,
- performance and assessment results,
- attendance and participation in treatment program or meeting with therapist (date and duration), and
- short-term treatment plans.

Discharge

Finally, the discharge summary and future plans are documented in a patient's final note. The discharge summary traditionally compares and contrasts the specific treatment goals with the progress made while under the care of the recreational therapist. Did the patient meet the respective goals? Are there remaining goals that are recommended for outpatient or future treatment through recommended channels? The therapist then documents future goals or recommendations regarding the patient's plans to maintain a healthy lifestyle.

Agency Protocols for Documentation

Although there are many general best practices for effective documentation, agencies establish specific protocols based on the needs of the patients they serve.

Agency Documentation Policies

Because each agency has clientele with different needs, the how, what, where, and when of documentation are often dictated by the specific agency. It is critical for the recreational therapist to be familiar with policies and protocols regarding documentation and charting within the respective agency. For example, how often a recreational therapist documents would depend on the agency. The frequency of documentation can occur per session, per day, per week, or even per quarter. For example, if therapeutic services are provided infrequently for the patient who resides at a facility and their health status remains unchanged for long periods of time, it might be appropriate for the RT to document monthly or quarterly. The regulatory requirements, frequency of treatment, and the variability of the patient's health status within the agency often dictate the documentation protocol. Burlingame and Blaschko (2010) suggested that therapists should document frequently enough to demonstrate continuity of care. Frequency of documentation protocol is also influenced at an agency by the amount of allocated staff time usage (Stumbo & Peterson, 2009).

Use of Abbreviations in Medical Charts

To expedite the documentation process, agencies will often adopt abbreviations for medical terms to help the therapist write a more efficient note (Skalko, 1998). Medical chart abbreviations are commonly used within paper charts and often incorporated into EMR computer platforms to assist the therapist in the charting process. Agencies commonly have an officially approved and adopted abbreviations list. It is important for recreational therapists to familiarize themselves with the agency's adopted list of approved medical abbreviations. Though not an exhaustive list, appendix A provides some common abbreviations used in health care settings.

Agency Adopted Formats

Although there are numerous formats for documentation, most agencies utilize a format designed for the specific setting and population. With today's electronic medical record keeping (EMR), agencies often dictate the format used for implementing the APIE process. Regardless of the agency or setting, formats generally utilize similar information. As noted by the Centers for Medicare and Medicaid Services (CMS):

> You should be aware that hospitals are increasingly using integrated databases, particularly in the areas of evaluations and treatment plans. Separate data collection is not a problem as long as it is integrated into multidisciplinary evaluations and treatment plans. (2015, p. 6)

Therefore, regardless of the setting or population, an agency should develop a coherent documentation plan that includes each discipline. It would be nearly impossible to explain the many different documentation formats and systems, so this chapter will explain some of the commonly used documentation systems used in health care in either paper-based or electronic charting formats.

Types of Documentation Systems

There are many different charting formats for documenting patient outcomes. As mentioned earlier, the type of documentation system adopted should be best suited to the needs of the agency and clientele. Three common documentation systems and subsequent formats within each system will be presented (i.e., free form, POMR, and alternate streamline systems).

Free Form Record Keeping

It is likely that the first format of medical charting was a documentation system called free form record keeping. This "system" isn't an actual system at all but a blank sheet for the therapist to document without any format or structure. This type of documentation system is the most basic form and tends to be more popular in more community-based service providers where other service providers do not need to review medical charts on a frequent basis. Because this system does not have a structure or organize content within a chart, it is difficult for others to efficiently locate specific content. One documentation format within this system is called *narrative* or *journaling*.

Narrative Progress Note Documentation

Narrative and journaling documentation is written in a simple story-telling paragraph format. The recreational therapist writes the narrative note in chronological order as events happen. The narrative note typically includes the date, body of the note, and the signature/credentials of the individual responsible for the content (Stumbo & Peterson, 2009). The skilled recreational therapist can still use narrative documentation to promote efficiencies for content and best practices. Figure 4.3 provides an example of a narrative note.

Advantages of Free Form Progress Notes

Because of their simplicity and limited structure, narrative documentation notes are easy for the practitioner to write. This simplicity also does not require extensive training for the therapist, therapy aide, or volunteer to assist in the documentation process. The practitioner does not have to determine where to put specific information or data. This format also allows space for the practitioner to provide extra details for explaining the data or events. Finally, writing events in the sequential order in which they occurred can also help the therapist in accurate memory recall.

Disadvantages of Free Form Progress Notes

Even though the lack of structure of the narrative note is easy to write, the lack of structure fails to provide direction for the content of the note and, if not careful, can become cumbersome and time consuming because the lack of

---

FIGURE 4.3   Example of a narrative progress note.

I.M. Pirate #19473, 4/24/19
Participant attended initial community RT play group on 4/20/19 with mother. Participant was
initially isol. from other group members but ↑ interactions after 15 minutes. Participant exhibits
issues c̄ normative developmental play skills for child her age including ability to sit ⓘ bilateral
UE fine motor grasp skills, and object permanence cognitive development. Participant will
benefit from continued therapeutic play group. Complete IA prior to next session and F/U c̄
mother to assess play skills demonstrated at home with older siblings.-------------------------------
Sam Therapist, CTRS

focus tends to cause the therapist to provide too many details (Quinn & Gordon, 2010). An even bigger disadvantage of the narrative progress note is that the lack of structure makes it difficult for other staff to utilize for communication.

Narrative progress notes require reading the entire note to learn more about a particular patient when another practitioner may only be interested in a specific piece of information. Despite some of the obvious disadvantages mentioned, the narrative progress note remains a simple documentation system that can be utilized in settings that do not require frequent team communication about the status of a patient. Problem-oriented progress notes, however, provide sectional categories for other practitioners to locate important information regarding the treatment of an individual.

Problem-Oriented Medical Records (POMR)

Problem-oriented medical record keeping is a format that categorizes the medical chart into various sections to focus on different types of problems (Stumbo & Peterson, 2009). This type of documentation system was developed as a way to better organize the patient's chart to make it easier for the reader. A classic study comparing the narrative versus the problem-oriented method found that "Nurses who applied the problem-oriented method of charting did record more pertinent information than those nurses who recorded in the traditional manner (Bertucci, Huston, & Perloff, 1974, p. 351).

There are many benefits of the POMR system, including the primary instrument of intra- and inter-provider communication among health care providers, accountability, billing, and legal and liability issues (Springhouse, 1999). The most common problem-oriented documentation system is the SOAP note.

SOAP Note Format

The SOAP note format was developed by Dr. Lawrence Weed in the 1960s (Weed, 1964). There have been recent debates whether the SOAP note is still relevant or needed even more in today's health care (Jeroudi & Payne, 2019). Despite mixed opinions, it remains one of the oldest and most commonly used charting formats today. Dr. Weed, a medical educator, developed the SOAP format to help teach medical students the art of collecting patient signs in four problem-oriented categories, including subjective, objective, assessment, and plan (Pearce, Ferguson, George, & Langford, 2016).

Subjective (S)   The subjective (S) section includes patient self-reported items, pertinent patient quotes related to health status, and family-reported information (Quinn & Gordon, 2010). Information documented in the S section of the SOAP note includes things that are not observed (see figure 4.4). Patient quotes are indicated by quotation marks (" "). It is also recommended that contextual clarification be provided for quotes that may require identification of the relevance to the patient's health condition. Because the S section of the SOAP note is subjective and often not verifiable, it is often seen as the least significant section of the SOAP note. Therefore, the recreational therapist should only include an S entry if it is significant to the patient's health status. If there isn't an entry, it is common to place a "Ø" to indicate that an entry was not applicable.

FIGURE 4.4   Example of SOAP subjective (S) section.

| I.M. Pirate |
| #19473 |

4/24/19

S: "I don't need all these therapists. I'm going to be walking tomorrow." (re: patient's denial

concerning complete SCI).--

Leaving the line blank might indicate to the reader that the section was neglected.

Objective (O)   The next section of the SOAP note, objective (O), was designed to report data that is verified and observable by the therapist. These items include the therapist's observations and treatment interventions utilized to treat the patient. One important insertion in O should always be documentation that treatment was provided. The entry should include the date, duration, and intervention. For example, the entry might include "CTRS provided 30-minute endurance training session on (date)." Best practices would encourage the recreational therapist to document the interventions in the O section first to avoid forgetting the entry. In this section, the therapist should avoid behavioral descriptions that do not include observable physical or behavioral symptoms. Words such as *sad*, *happy*, or *mad* should be avoided unless supported with physical or behavioral evidence the therapist used to make such determinations. For example, a more appropriate O entry would indicate "the patient expressed anger as demonstrated by his elevated volume and obscene language." Figure 4.5 provides an example of the O section.

Assessment (A)   The third section of the SOAP note is assessment (A), in which the therapist is provided the opportunity to analyze, synthesize, and provide clinical impressions of the patient's condition (Burlingame & Blaschko, 2010). The A section (see figure 4.6) is the only section of the SOAP note that provides the recreational therapist the opportunity to expand upon their clinical views and analysis based on the S and O sections. Did the patient meet their goals this week? Is the patient progressing or regressing based on the particular reporting period? Justification of future plans in the P section are often made in the A section. For example, the recreational therapist may record, "The patient will benefit from continued participation in the exercise group to increase strength and endurance to promote further mobility independence and goal attainment in other therapies."

Plan (P)   The final section, plan (P), is where the recreational therapist indicates *how* the treatment will be developed and implemented to reach the patient's goals or objectives (see figure 4.7). There is certainly a connection between the assessment (A) and the plan (P), because the P section provides the proposed strategies to address the diagnoses listed in A. Whether listed or in a more narrative provision, the P section provides the primary therapist, or those covering for the therapist, specific strategies for the treatment of the patient.

FIGURE 4.5   Example of SOAP objective (O) section.

O: Referral received on 4/21/19 for RT services. Pt. met with RT for 30 minute IA. Pt is a 75

yo female African-American. Dx of Ⓛ CVA with some impaired function on Ⓡ Pre-morbid

hx indicates mod. activity level with min. cognitive issues. Tx team reports some memory

and mobility issues. Pt. presented with positive affect and receptiveness to RT services.-----

---

FIGURE 4.6   Example of SOAP assessment (A) section.

A: Pt. is increasing w/c mobility on community outings but will benefit from continued outings

to ↑ advanced barrier management skills including curbs, doors, and rough terrain. Pt remains

focused on ↑ UE strength for continued Ⓘ Pt requires additional aquatic Tx for balance

and endurance.--

FIGURE 4.7   Example of SOAP plan (P) section.

P: 1) Complete IA c̄ pt., 2) F/U c̄ family to confirm post-D/C resources. 3) Schedule meeting
    c̄ peer support group to ↑ motivation.--

Modified Versions of the SOAP Note

Since the inception and adoption of the SOAP note format, there have been many modified versions that include structured sections that align with the provider's setting. The following are examples of common formats adapted from the original SOAP note format.

SOAPIER Chart Format

Over the years, modification of the traditional SOAP note has evolved (Jeroudi & Payne, 2019). For example, the SOAPIER note was developed to provide an extension to the original four charting categories provided in Dr. Lawrence Weed's SOAP note.

   Subjective: What the patient says
   Objective: What you observed
   Assessment: Assessment or analysis
   Plan: What you plan to do to correct this problem

Implementation: Intervention or action that you performed

Evaluation: Patient response to the treatment

Revision: Any changes needed or made to the implementation

Behavioral Intervention Response Plan (BIRP) Notes

Another modified version of the SOAP note is the Behavioral Intervention Response Plan (BIRP) note. The BIRP note is similar to the SOAP note in terms of structure, except that it has sections that relate more to psychiatric or behavioral health settings and approaches (Austin, 2013). The BIRP sections (see figure 4.8) are described here.

Behavior (B)   The B section of the note describes the behavior relevant to the target health outcome of the patient in behavioral health or psychiatric settings. Some typical descriptions might include *withdrawn, hyperac-*

FIGURE 4.8   Example of BIRP progress note.

	I.M. Pirate
	#19473

4/24/19

B:	"I don't have a drinking problem. I can quit drinking anytime I need to." (re: patient's denial concerning ETOH addiction). Pt. Dx ETOH addiction.---
I:	Referral received on 4/21/19 for RT services. Pt. met with RT for 30 minute IA. IA indicates Pt. has hx of ETOH use and has 6 DUI citations. Pt. provided 1:1 session and overview of RT services.---
R:	Pt. presented with pleasant affect but verbalized initial resistance to Tx due to denial of addiction.---
P:	1) Complete IA & ITP, 2) schedule group x2, 3) monitor side effects of ETOH withdrawal.----

Sam Therapist, CTRS

tive, task-oriented, impulsive, friendly, interactive w/peers, angry, assertive, aggressive, sad, tearful, despondent, clingy, needy, attention seeking, well-mannered, polite, calm, jovial, or *anxious.*

Intervention (I)   The I section of the BIRP note describes the therapist's intervention used to address the target health outcome. Examples of these interventions may include approaches such as problem solving, conflict resolution, behavior management, stress management, group discussion therapy, deep breathing, coping skills, social skills groups, and other psychosocial and behavioral health approaches. Like the SOAP note, this section should also document the patient's participation in the intervention or treatment provided with the date and duration of participation.

Response (R)   The R section is the response of the patient to the therapist's intervention. Was the patient receptive or resistant to the approach? Did they complete therapeutic exercises as requested in group setting? Did they demonstrate an understanding of the therapeutic approach? This section is the therapist's interpretation of the reaction of the patient.

Plan (P)   The P section provides the therapist's plan for the treatment of the individual. Much of this section relates to the next approach with the patient, including continuing to assess, monitor, support, educate, encourage, or discharge.

Advantages of Problem-Oriented Medical Records (POMR)

Today, there are many different formats of the original POMR, the SOAP note. SOAP notes are one of the oldest and most recognized documentation formats in health care (Quinn & Gordon, 2010). This universal acceptance has created a general familiarity across health care (Austin, 2013). Even some EMR incorporate versions of the SOAP note within digital templates (Pearce et al., 2016). Another advantage of POMR systems is promotion of team communication. Because entries are segmented into categories, the ability to locate information in the chart is quick and efficient. For example, if a recreational therapist is covering for

another therapist on vacation, they can easily review the previous week's SOAP note to determine what was completed (O), review therapist impressions on the current status of the patient (A), and easily identify the plan to continue (P).

Disadvantages of Problem-Oriented Medical Records (POMR)

While one of the oldest and most familiar documentation systems in use, there may be some disadvantages of POMR systems. First, POMR systems often promote documentation that is too concise, with limited opportunities to explain if the entry does not fit into one of the categories. Another criticism of POMR systems is that they routinely overuse abbreviations, acronyms, and medical jargon that is difficult for the nonprofessional to decipher. The Health Insurance Portability and Accountability Act of 1996 (HIPAA) mandates individuals receiving care have more access to their medical records. According to HIPAA:

> *The Privacy Rule generally requires HIPAA covered entities (health plans and most health care providers) to provide individuals, upon request, with access to the protected health information (PHI) about them in one or more "designated record sets" maintained by or for the covered entity. This includes the right to inspect or obtain a copy, or both, of the PHI, as well as to direct the covered entity to transmit a copy to a designated person or entity of the individual's choice. (HHS, 2019)*

Individuals have the right to access their personal health information (PHI) in a "designated record set" which is defined at 45 CFR 164.501 as medical records, billing records, or other records used to make decisions about an individual's health care. This new legislation may provide future trends toward reduced use of medical jargon and abbreviations so the treated individual can read and understand their own care pathway. Finally, some have also suggested that POMR systems tend to be too linear and sequential. Delitto and Snyder-Mackler (1995) suggested POMR systems encourage a sequential rather than integrative approach to clinical reasoning, and there is often a tendency for the health professional to merely collect information, not *assess* and *interpret* it.

Alternate Streamline Documentation Systems

Finally, there are a variety of alternate streamline documentation systems in health care. Some systems limit entries to only documenting out-of-the-ordinary events or only routine treatments. Because these systems *only* document the routine care or *only* occurrences outside of normative care, they are often much more efficient than typical problem-oriented documentation. The following section of this chapter provides alternate systems that document care that is *only* routine or a variance from the norm.

Focus Charting (DAR) Format

One of the criticisms of the narrative charting format is that it is difficult to find specific entries because they are not organized into retrievable sections. Stumbo and Peterson (2009) suggested that the focus charting format is a way to organize such narrative entries by placing content into columns. Each entry is concentrated around a focus or specific outcome, patient concern, behavior, or a significant change in a patient's status. The columns of the focus charting note (see figure 4.9) include the following:

- *Date/time.* Column 1 of the focus chart includes the date and time the note was written. The date includes the month, day, and year (e.g., 03/27/2019) and the time is typically provided in military time to prevent confusion (e.g., "1400" to indicate 2:00 p.m.).

- *Focus.* The second column is the focus of the progress note. This often includes things like a patient's diagnostic problem (e.g., depression, obesity), acute changes in patient's health status (e.g., seizures, bed-ridden), significant events in treatment (e.g., community reintegration outing), or compliance with RT standard of care (e.g., RT treatment plan). With the growth in use of the ICF, the focus area is often provided with the specific ICF code. For example, a focus for an individual who lacks balance might include b2351, vestibular function of balance, in the "Focus" column.

- *Note.* The third column includes the body of the progress note. The body of the note is further categorized into data (D), action (A), response (R), and sometimes plan (P). Each section includes the following content:

  ○ Data (D): Subjective and objective entries that support the focus or describe the status of the patient at the time of a significant event or intervention

---

FIGURE 4.9   Example of focus charting (DAR) format.

Client: | I.M. Pirate #19473

Date/Time	Focus	D = Data A = Action R = Response P = Plan
04/13/2019 1300	Vestibular Balance b2351	D: Ind. 30 min. IA. A: TUG administered. R: TUG score 10.7 seconds. Time greater than normative range for 60 yo but well below cut-off value predictive of falls. P: Initiate Matter of Balance program. Monitor progress and reassess in 1 month.

Staff: | Sam Therapist, CTRS

- Action (A): Completed or planned interventions (e.g., group therapy, stress management, one-on-one follow-up with therapist) to address the stated focus area
- Response (R): Description of the patient's response to intervention and progress in achieving goals
- Plan (P): Description of short-term interventions to be implemented

Focus or DAR notes do not need to always have a plan (P) section. They do not even need to have all three DAR sections. Some focus chart notes may contain one or two of the three parts. Only relevant entries need to be included. Figure 4.9 provides a sample of a focus (DAR) note. Many supporters of the focus/DAR progress note contend that the focus is much more encompassing than the problem incorporated in the POMR system (Stumbo & Peterson, 2009).

Clinical Flow Sheets

Health care is often an endless cycle of routine treatment provided to a patient. The documentation of such routine care becomes tiresome and monotonous, requiring the creation of a format to document these tasks, called a clinical flow sheet. Flow sheets are quick, view-at-a-glance sheets, typically one or two pages, that list routine tasks provided by the therapist or reactions by the patient. Rather than writing a narrative entry, the therapist typically has the option of checking a box that indicates they or the patient performed the routine task. Flow sheets are often supplemental with more narrative documentation formats. Items documented within the flow sheet do not need to be repeated in the narrative note. The flow sheet also serves as a reminder, or check sheet, for the therapist to complete basic routine care as part of the treatment protocol (Quinn & Gordon, 2010). Flow sheets are more commonly used in nursing care where a practitioner might document certain vital signs (e.g., temperature, appetite, weight) over a certain period of time. Recreational therapists may also utilize flow sheets to indicate and document certain goals for patients. Flow sheets may also be organized in such a manner that they indicate participation or nonparticipation in treatment groups when common expectations are anticipated. The efficiency of flow sheets and easy access and communication to team members remains a vital reason for the popularity of this format. However, flow sheets can only be used for routine tasks expected of all treatments.

Clinical Pathways

Another concept related to the documentation of routine care and flow sheets is the use of clinical pathways. *Clinical pathways* are evidence-based road maps that assist in reducing variations in clinical practice (Hipp, Abel, & Weber, 2016). These "road maps" are preestablished guidelines and protocols in the management of a specific diagnostic group. For example, a 70-year-old female with a right hip replacement would have a clinical pathway with flow sheets that establish how her care is managed, how quickly she should progress, and a protocol for the treatment of her medical problem.

Charting by Exception (CBE) or Variance Charting

The final alternate streamline documentation system is charting by exception (CBE). CBE, or variance charting, is a charting format wherein the therapist documents those items within the clinical pathway and expands upon *exceptions* to those pathways (i.e., charting by exception). When a patient is progressing along the expected pathway for their diagnostic grouping, the therapist checks a box or initials a certain level indicating the routine care or predetermined progress was completed. If the patient demonstrates a variance from the predetermined pathway, then a CBE note is written. This format of documentation tends to be more efficient, because the routine care is indicated on the flow sheet and only variances from the standard pathway are further explained with the date, intended outcome, explanation of why variance occurred, and plan to address variance (Smith, 2002).

Advantages of Alternate Streamline Documentation Charting

The focus chart, flow sheet, and charting by exception formats all provide quick and efficient charting because documentation is limited to only addressing specific outcomes, routine care, or variances from preestablished pathways. Because these formats are streamlined, the therapist tends to spend less time on paperwork and charting and more time with direct patient contact (Smith, 2002). Furthermore, these formats often enhance consistency because the system establishes standards and protocols that reduce individual variations in documentation quality and quantity. They also often emphasize and highlight variances in care that require change or a patient's status from the norm indicating a clear need for intervention. Alternate documentation systems that only focus on routine care or exceptions provide health care providers specific reference points that can more easily be read and understood, which ultimately enhances continuity of care. Finally, preestablished care guidelines and clinical pathways within flow sheets become easy references and reminders, reducing the risk of inadvertent deviation from the standard of treatment.

Disadvantages of Alternate Streamline Documentation Charting

At face value, these focused and streamlined systems seem like the answer to the ever-challenging issue of time-consuming and cumbersome documentation. However, there are some concerns regarding the use of these documentation systems. First, many of these systems are based on pathways or preestablished routine care. The development of these protocols must be proven through evidence-based analysis that can take enormous amounts of time. Smith (2002) also suggested that these streamlined systems should be eval-uated before adoption to ensure there isn't a conflict with state and federal regulations or those of accreditation agencies such as the Joint Commission (TJC) (formerly the Joint Commission on Accreditation of Healthcare Organizations [JCAHO]). Agency personnel, including risk managers and facility attorneys, will need to review and approve adoption of such streamlined documentation systems so as not to put the agency at risk for potential lawsuits. Heron (2014) suggested that these limited documentation systems could be a trap for poor documentation and potential negligence. These predetermined care pathways can be effective if and only if they are based on clearly defined standards of practice and predetermined criteria for assessments and interventions. When agency definitions are incomplete, vague, or poorly designed, the variance or exception may be overlooked and patients may be at risk. Heron (2014) further criticized this "one size fits all" approach, which may suggest a "normal" finding in the definitions is abnormal for another patient (Heron, 2014). Certainly, these types of streamlined systems may be a potential solution for the documentation workload, but some have indicated they could come at a very significant cost to patient care.

Digital Documentation

Much of this chapter has discussed the debate of paper-based versus digital or online documentation. This chapter was not meant to answer such a debate. However, one thing that is not debatable is the fact that the adoption of electronic health records (EHR) or electronic medical records (EMR) is growing exponentially and the recreational therapist needs to be prepared to document in the digital world. The Health Information Technology for Economic and Clinical Health (HITECH) Act was passed in 2009, increasing the use of EMR in health care. The HITECH Act used financial incentives to promote increased adoption of digital documentation among health care agencies. Charles, King, Patel, and Furukawa (2013) suggested that since the passing of the HITECH Act, the percentage of agencies adopting EMR tripled from 2009 to 2013.

Benefits of EMR

Quinn and Gordon (2010) suggested there are many benefits to adopting EMR systems. First, the use of EMR standardizes data elements and charting protocols because all individuals are using the same system. EMR systems also provide the health care provider real time access to patient data. Legibility of data entries is also improved through the use of electronic data entry, and only agency-approved medical abbreviations are embedded within adopted EMR systems. In addition, standardized assessments like the Functional Independence Measure (FIM), via *FIMWare*, can be incorporated into systems to expedite assessment and documentation workflow (Quinn & Gordon, 2010). The use of EMR also eliminates the need for massive storage space for paper-based records. Martinez Monterrubio and colleagues (2015) suggested that EMR practices improve confidentiality and reduce fraud of the medical record with built-in security measures.

While the benefits of EMR are worthy in and of themselves, the most critical purpose of electronic documentation is the hope that it will decrease the amount of time health care providers spend documenting (Wang, 2012). Clinch and Kellet (2015) suggested that clinicians spend 25 to 50 percent of their time completing documentation. The goal of EMR systems is to use standardized documentation templates that expedite the documentation process.

EMR Templates

Many of the documentation systems discussed in this chapter can be provided in an electronic template. The template provides a chart in one page that allows the therapist to utilize the various software functionality to record, save, and transmit notes in a single entry. Other traditional functions of EMR platforms include fill-in-the-blank fields, customized preprogrammed options, instant access to the entire database of EMR for historical review, and customized shortcuts to fit the preferences of each therapist. Many of the EMR platforms also allow the agency to customize their own templates so that the agency workflow matches the system capacity. There are hundreds of companies specializing in EMR systems, so learning how to use the system is agency-centric.

Criticism of EMR

While there are many benefits of EMR, there are some criticisms and cautionary advice in the universal adoption. While the most important benefit of EMR is certainly efficiency, some have suggested that the incredible learning curve to become proficient with each new system adds more time and burden to an already overworked health care provider (Baumann, Baker, & Elshaug, 2018). Baumann and colleagues examined time spent in documentation after EMR adoption and found that physicians' documentation time *increased* from 16 to 28 percent and nurses from 9 to 23 percent. This significant learning curve has caused mixed attitudes among health care practitioners toward adopting EMR as a routine practice (Clinch & Kellet, 2015).

Another stated benefit of EMR systems is the accuracy of notes. Although some individuals suggest that EMR reduces redundancy and errors (Quinn & Gordon, 2010), Weng (2017) suggested that electronic charts often contain more errors than expected despite claims from technology companies that the systems are nearly error-proof. Weir and colleagues (2003) conducted an audit of medical charts in the Veteran's Health Administration's EMR and found that 60 percent of progress notes contained at least one documentation error (mean = 7.8 documentation errors per chart). Weiss and Levy (2014) suggested that the biggest concern to errors in EMR is the common practice of copying and transferring data from one patient to another. They suggested in a chart analysis study that mistakes in copying and pasting contributed to 35.7 percent of errors in electronic charting. This common practice of copying and pasting from other sections of the patient's chart or even from other patients entirely is called *chart cloning*. Cloning has become a current and critical risk in documentation today (Weiss & Levy, 2014) that has produced errors that led to the denial of Medicare payments due to medical fraud (Cueva, 2019). The recreational therapist should continue to use good common documentation practices when using EMR to avoid such risks.

Promoting Good Habits With EMR

EMR is a technological tool developed to assist the therapist with documentation. However, this form of technology was never meant to replace the therapist's knowledge base and critical thinking in the documentation process (Pearce et al., 2016). Weiss and Levy (2014) provided some best practice recommendations for using EMR:

- The final author is responsible for all content of the signed progress note.

- The person responsible for the progress note should review and update all copied or otherwise imported information meticulously.

- Any information copied and pasted should be clearly identified with quotes, italics, or different fonts to indicate information was copied.

- All EMR notes should include attribution of source (date, time, and original author) in copied text or data.

- Data copied or imported should be essential and pertinent to the clinical encounter.

- Agencies should invest financial and time resources to fully educate staff to create high-quality documentation with EMR tools.

Future Issues in Documentation

Health care is a rapidly changing market and documentation is sure to evolve in the future. For example, new HIPAA laws provide patients more privacy and personal accessibility to their own medical records. The old way of documentation will certainly not be understood by the nonmedical layperson reading their own notes. Some have suggested that health care providers will soon need to do away with the typical medical jargon embedded in charts so that care providers *and* patients can understand the contents of medical charts (Wang, 2012).

Furthermore, technology will continue to be both an asset and challenge to health care providers. Technology changes so quickly that it is often outdated as soon as it is out of the box. EMR will be universally adopted in the future as new technologies continue to make documentation more efficient and accessible. For example, point-of-care documentation is becoming common as more therapists incorporate tablets to provide documentation as care is provided (Weng, 2017). This will allow immediate recording to prevent memory decay and improve efficiency to reduce documentation workload. The future is filled with many new technologies that aim to find the most accurate and efficient mechanisms for the recreational therapist and other allied health providers.

Summary

The use of accurate and compliant patient documentation is an essential skill for all recreational therapy professionals. Agencies will typically have their own established methods and formats for documentation. It is incumbent upon the developing recreational therapist to become familiar with the agency's processes, preferred charting abbreviations, and desired practices.

This chapter offers sound general guidelines that are relatively congruent with most health care settings. It is incumbent on the recreational therapy preprofessional and professional to integrate appropriate practices that are compliant with all regulatory agencies, including the Centers for Medicare and Medicaid Services (CMS), State Department of Health Services (DHS), the Joint Commission (TJC), and the Commission on Accreditation of Rehabilitation Facilities (CARF).

REFLECTION QUESTIONS

1. In your own words, write at least one paragraph describing the role of the Centers for Medicare and Medicaid Services (CMS) with regard to agency compliance and the assessment process.
2. Describe how the documentation fits into the APIE process at each phase.
3. Describe each part of a SOAP note.
4. Give one example of a SMART goal for each of the following ICF codes:

    d160

    d175

    d7104

    d4452
5. Identify at least four key guidelines for writing progress notes (e.g., date and sign).

REFERENCES

American Therapeutic Recreation Association (ATRA). (2013). *Standards for the practice of recreational therapy.* Hattiesburg, MS: American Therapeutic Recreation Association.

Austin, L. (2013). Treatment planning and case management in community mental health. In D. Maller (Ed.), *The Praeger handbook of community mental health practice* (pp. 83-102). Santa Barbara, CA: Praeger.

Baumann, L.A., Baker, J., & Elshaug, A.G. (2018). The impact of electronic health record systems on clinical documentation times: A systematic review. *Health Policy, 122,* 827-836.

Bertucci, M., Huston, M., & Perloff, E. (1974). Comparative study of progress notes using problem-oriented and traditional methods of charting. *Nursing Research, 23*(4), 351-354.

Bexelius, A., Carlberg, E.B., & Lowing, K. (2018). Quality of goal setting in pediatric rehabilitation—A SMART approach. *Child: Care, Health, and Development, 44*(6), 850-856.

Burlingame, J., & Blaschko, T.M. (2010). *Assessment tools for recreational therapy and related fields* (4th ed.). Ravensdale, WA: Idyll Arbor.

Centers for Medicare and Medicaid Services (CMS). (2015). *State operations manual for psychiatric hospitals—Interpretive guidelines and survey procedures (Rev. 149, 10-09-15) Transmittals for appendix AA part I—Investigative procedures survey protocol—Psychiatric hospitals.* Retrieved from www.cms.gov/Regulations-and-Guidance/Guidance/Manuals/Downloads/som107ap_aa_psyc_hospitals.pdf

Charles, D., King, J., Patel, V., & Furukawa, M.F. (2013). *ONC Data Brief No. 9: Adoption of electronic health record systems among US non-federal acute care hospitals: 2008-2012.* Washington, DC: Office of the National Coordinator for Health Information Technology. Retrieved from http://healthitgov-stage.ahrqstg.org

Charney, P. (2012, Dec.). Electronic medical records: Are nutrition support professionals ready? *Nutrition in Clinical Practice, 27*(6), 715-717.

Clinch, N., & Kellett, J. (2015). Medical documentation: Part of the solution, or part of the problem? A narrative review of the literature on the time spent on and value of medical documentation. *International Journal of Medical Informatics, 84*(4), 221-228.

Cueva, J.P. (2019). EMR cloning: A bad habit. *Chicago Medical Society.* Retrieved from www.cmsdocs.org/news/emr-cloning-a-bad-habit

Delitto, A., & Snyder-Mackler, L. (1995). The diagnostic process: Examples in orthopedic physical therapy. *Physical Therapy, 75*(3), 203-211.

Department of Health and Human Services (HHS). (2019). Health information privacy: Individuals' right under HIPAA to access their health information, 45 CFR § 164.524. Retrieved from www.hhs.gov/hipaa/for-professionals/privacy/guidance/access/index.html

Heron, J. (2014, Feb.). Charting by exception: A trap for poor documentation. *Med League.* Retrieved from www.medleague.com/charting-by-exceptiona-expert-witness

Hipp, R., Abel, E., & Weber, R.J. (2016). Director's forum: A primer on clinical pathways. *Hospital Pharmacy, 51*(5), 416-421.

Jeroudi, S., & Payne, J.D. (2019). Remembering Lawrence Weed: A pioneer of the SOAP note to the editor. *Academic Medicine, 94*(1), 11.

Martinez Monterrubio, S.M., Juan, F.S., & Raúl, M.B. (2015). EMR log method for computer security for electronic medical records with logic and data mining. *BioMed Research International*, 1-12.

Pearce, P.F., Ferguson, L.A., George, G.S., & Langford, C.A. (2016). The essential SOAP note in an EHR era. *The Nurse Practitioner, 2*, 29-36.

Quinn, L., & Gordon, J. (2010). *Documentation for rehabilitation - E-book: A guide to clinical decision making* (2nd ed.). St. Louis, MO: Saunders (Elsevier Science).

Skalko, T.K. (1998). *Medical abbreviations for the health professions*. Ravensdale, WA: Idyll Arbor.

Smith, L.S. (2002). How to chart by exception. *Nursing, 32*(9), 30.

Springhouse Corp. (1999). *Mastering documentation* (2nd ed.). Springhouse, PA: Springhouse Publishing.

Stumbo, N.J. (2003). *Patient assessment in therapeutic recreation services*. Urbana, IL: Sagamore.

Stumbo, N.J., & Peterson, C.A. (2009). *Therapeutic recreation program design: Principles and procedures* (5th ed.). Urbana, IL: Sagamore-Venture.

Wang, C.J. (2012). Medical documentation in the electronic era. *JAMA, 308*(20), 2091-2092.

Weed, L.L. (1964). Medical records, patient care, and medical education. *Irish Journal of Medical Science, 462*, 271-282.

Weir, C.R., Hurdle, J.F., Felgar, M.A., Hoffman, J.M., Roth, B., & Nebeker, J.R. (2003). Direct text entry in electronic progress notes: An evaluation of input errors. *Methods of Information in Medicine, 42*(1), 61-67.

Weiss, J.W., & Levy, P.C. (2014). Copy, paste, and cloned notes in electronic health records: Prevalence, benefits, risks, and best practice recommendations. *CHEST-Topics in Practice Management, 140*(3), 632-638.

Weng, C.Y. (2017). Data accuracy in electronic medical record documentation. *JAMA Ophthalmology, 135*(3), 232-233.

Wilkinson, J., Treas, L., & Barnett, K. (2015). *Fundamentals of nursing (two volume set)*. Retrieved from https://ebookcentral.proquest.com

World Health Organization. (2001). *ICF: International classification of functioning, disability and health*. Geneva: Author.

CHAPTER 5

Assessment and Aging: Considerations and Recommendations for Recreational Therapy

Megan C. Janke, PhD, LRT/CTRS

Marieke Van Puymbroeck, PhD, CTRS, FDRT

LEARNING OBJECTIVES

Upon completion of the text, the student will demonstrate:

- Knowledge of evidence-based recreational therapy assessment instruments used to determine physical, cognitive, emotional, and social functioning of older adults.

- Knowledge of the evidence of problems and limitations that may occur in an older adult population.

- Knowledge of evidence-based assessment instruments from other health care disciplines that may be relevant to recreational therapy practice when assessing older adults.

- Knowledge of the World Health Organization's (WHO) *International Classification of Functioning, Disability and Health* (ICF) as a method of classifying individual functioning and the impact of activity limitations and restrictions to participation in life activities, independence, satisfaction, and quality of life.

If we are lucky, we will all experience the aging process. However, society has a variety of perspectives about the process. Aging is often seen as negative and fraught with disease, infirmity, and cognitive impairment. While those issues can occur at any age, simply growing older does not mean that comorbidities will exist. However, stereotypes of the aging process can influence how recreational therapists (and other clinicians) treat their older clients. These stereotypes are addressed in the next section and should be taken into consideration as the assessment process is undertaken. There are further considerations that the recreational therapist should take into account when preparing to do an assessment with an older adult, such as the potential for the presence of hearing impairments, orthostatic hypotension, and delirium and dementia. This chapter concludes with a description of various assessment resources and specific tools that may be appropriate for use with older adults. This section includes the corresponding ICF code for easy reference.

Stereotypes of Aging and the Assessment Process

We all have stereotypes that affect our interactions with the people and world around us. When working with older adults, it is critical to be mindful of our personal stereotypes of the aging population, because this might affect our approach to the assessment process. Take a moment to think about some of the stereotypes related to older adults that are prevalent in our society. Remember that stereotypes are not inherently negative or positive, but rather refer to a widely accepted belief or image of a particular group. Some of the common stereotypes about the aging population include characteristics such as frail, hard of hearing, unwilling to try new things, or poor drivers. They could also include more positive attributes such as wise, caring, and supportive. While these descriptions are true for some older adults, they do not apply to all aging individuals. This is important to keep in mind because these stereotypes have the potential to influence our

expectations and even evaluations of an aging client's performance. The ability of attitudes to affect individual behavior and social life is categorized as negative or discriminatory practices in the ICF (e410-e499).

Ageism is a common concern for health care professionals and has the potential to affect how they treat and interact with this population (e450) (e.g., Higashi, Tillack, Steinman, Harper, & Johnson, 2012; McKenzie & Brown, 2014). Older adults themselves often have negative stereotypes that influence their own performance based on the acceptance of societal attitudes (e460) about aging. Research has found that negative stereotypes about age affect older adults' competence, particularly in areas related to cognitive performance (Lamont, Swift, & Abrams, 2015), and it can influence their perspective of their functional abilities as well. Recreational therapists need to make a conscious effort not to reinforce negative stereotypes during their assessment process. Do not make assumptions about an individual's physical ability to complete a functional assessment (e.g., balance, gait test) or cognitive assessment (e.g., memory/recall) based solely on their age. Challenge these stereotypes and encourage older adults to try to perform these assessments when there is no medical-related reason why they should not or could not complete them. Do not assume that an older individual has impaired physical functioning or cognitive capacity—and allow them to do as much as possible during the assessment process to safely gain a more comprehensive and accurate depiction of their abilities.

Other stereotypes that society has regarding older adults affect perceptions of their preferred leisure activities and hobbies (d920, e465). As recreational therapists, it is important for us to understand our clients' interests and gain a better understanding of their preferred activities during our assessments. Common perceptions of older adults' leisure often include activities such as bingo, watching TV, and sitting on the front porch, among other activities. It is important to remember that stereotypes emerge because they "fit" with a portion of a population, or did at one time. However, as recreational therapists, it is critical that we go into the assessment process with no preconceived ideas about the hobbies and interests of our clients based solely on their age. Older patients also engage in leisure activities attributed much less often to this population, such as competitive sports, sexual activity, or illicit drug use. Their preferred activities may be important to acknowledge and address in their treatment and can help with the identification of interventions that would be the most effective for them personally.

Factors That Influence Assessment in Older Adults

As previously noted, chronic conditions, and often several conditions at the same time, are very prevalent among older adults. This potentially leads to some issues during assessments that might not be common when working with other populations in recreational therapy. In this section, a few health-related and environmental factors will be identified and discussed as they relate to gathering accurate assessment data from aging clients. Understanding these aspects is important to ensure that our RT assessments are valid. If we do not take these factors into consideration, it is quite possible that our assessment results would be invalid or misleading, and thus might lead to the planning and implementation of inappropriate or ineffective interventions and treatment for the client.

Hearing Impairment

Nearly 25 percent of individuals aged 65 to 74 and 50 percent of individuals who are 75 and older have disabling hearing loss (NIDCD, 2016). Many of the assessments used in recreational therapy require older clients to understand and respond appropriately to different prompts (e.g., cognitive assessments, physical function assessments). Despite how common hearing loss is in the aging population, it is often underrecognized and undertreated (Yueh, Shapiro, MacLean, & Shekelle, 2003), in

part because the loss may occur so gradually that even the older adult does not realize the extent of their hearing impairment. However, this is a factor that therapists need to consider when conducting assessments with aging clients.

It is critical that practitioners make sure that an older adult's poor performance on a measurement is not due to their inability to clearly hear and understand the questions, rather than an actual low level of functioning in that domain (e.g., cognition, psychological well-being). A study by Lin (2011) suggested that greater hearing loss is associated with poorer performance on cognitive tests; however, hearing aid use is positively associated with cognitive functioning. This same study also indicated that the reduction in cognitive performance associated with a 25dB hearing loss was equivalent to the reduction in hearing associated with a client seven years older. If a client has hearing aids, it is critical that the therapist makes sure the client is using them for the assessment. For clients that might have unilateral hearing deficits (i.e., hearing loss that only affects one ear), the therapist should make sure that they are sitting in a position where the patient is best able to hear the instructions and questions that are being asked during the interview and assessment.

Orthostatic Hypotension

The medical condition orthostatic hypotension might also lead to some challenges when conducting assessments with the aging population. *Orthostatic hypotension* refers to a decrease in blood pressure by at least 20 mmHg in diastolic blood pressure or 10 mmHg in systolic blood pressure when transitioning from supine or sitting to standing. This condition becomes much more common as individuals age. It is thought to occur in approximately 10 to 30 percent of older adults who live at home (Rubenstein, 2006) but is more common among adults who reside in institutionalized settings such as nursing homes, possibly affecting almost 60 to 70 percent of residents (Figueroa, Basford, & Low, 2010; Weiss, Grossman, Beloosesky, & Grinblat, 2002). This condition may make some assessments difficult for recreational therapists to conduct because it is associated with dizziness, light-headedness, blurry vision, fainting, and even confusion. There have been some concerns raised about the increased potential for falls in adults with orthostatic hypotension, although research on this topic is mixed (Lipsitz, 2017). Recreational therapists need to be aware of the potential for orthostatic hypotension before conducting assessments with clients, particularly if these assessments require the patient to transfer quickly from lying down or seated to standing.

Medications

Older adults are more likely to be taking medications, especially multiple medications, than younger individuals. A survey of Medicare patients found that two out of five adults reported taking five or more prescription medications on a regular basis (Wilson, Schoen, Neuman, Strollo, Rogers, Chang, et al., 2007). This is a concern among the aging population due the potential side effects of these medications, and the fact that older adults are at a greater risk for drug interactions due to polypharmacy (taking multiple medications at one time). Some of the specific side effects that have been associated with medication use for older adults include falls, depression, confusion, hallucinations, and malnutrition (Murray & Callahan, 2003). As recreational therapists, it is important to understand the potential of medications and medication interactions to cause some of these negative outcomes in the aging population and realize that this may affect the validity of assessment outcomes. In addition, it is also critical to understand potential side effects of medications in order to take appropriate safety precautions during assessments. For example, if a recreational therapist is using an assessment to measure an older adult's balance and gait, but the client is currently taking a medication that has been linked to an increased risk of falling, it might be appropriate to consult with other members of the treatment team such as physical therapy to assist or ensure that another staff member is present to reduce the potential risk of falling.

Testing Environment

Another factor to be considered during assessment of older adults is the environment where the measurement is being conducted. There are many potential causes of external noises in clinical settings, including loud air conditioners, heavy foot traffic in the hallways, conversations between other individuals in the facility or at the nursing station, noisy medical equipment and monitoring systems, or messages over a public announcement system that might make it difficult for the client to hear the therapist clearly. When this occurs, the likelihood of an invalid assessment or misleading results in an assessment increases. For example, if a loud air conditioner makes it hard for a client to hear you during the assessment, she might provide answers that lead you to believe she is confused or disoriented, when she actually just misunderstood the questions asked.

Some diagnoses of our clients as well as age-related changes in functioning increase the need for a quiet testing environment during assessments. For older adults with impaired hearing, it is critical that assessments are conducted in spaces that are quiet and that do not have a lot of external or environmental noise. This is also a factor to consider when working with individuals who have had some type of head injury (Carroll, Cassidy, Cancelliere, Côté, Hincapié, Kristman, et al., 2014) and stroke (McDowd, Filion, Pohl, Richards, & Stiers, 2003), as they may also have difficulties with attention and be more easily distracted by outside sounds. In addition, research (e.g., Weeks & Hasher, 2014) has noted that older adults in general have a decreased ability to ignore irrelevant information, making them particularly susceptible to negative effects on their cognitive performance when there are distractions in their environment. This can lead to delayed response times, decreased comprehension, disrupted problem solving, and decreased memory performance. Based on this research and information, recreational therapists should take into consideration the environment where they are conducting assessments on older patients to minimize the effect that external noise and distractions will have on the adults' functional performance.

Connection to the *International Classification of Functioning, Disability and Health*

The factors discussed previously are related to aspects of the ICF model (WHO, 2001). An individual's hearing may be affected by aspects of body structure (e.g., s240, s250, s260), with impairment being caused due to damage of the inner, middle, or external structure of the ear. It is relevant in body function (e.g., b1560, auditory perception; b230, hearing functions) and influenced by environmental factors (e.g., e125, e535), such as the use of hearing aids or other assistive technology to enhance sounds and improve adults' ability to communicate.

Medications fit within the domain of personal factors, in that clients may choose to use them—correctly or incorrectly—to reduce the impairment and limitations they experience as a result of a change in body function. Orthostatic hypotension (b4201) may result in symptoms such as nausea (b2403) and dizziness (b2401), which are described in the body functions of the ICF. The testing environment is addressed in the environmental factors section of the ICF, including aspects such as lighting (e240) and sound (e250). In addition, all of the factors described in this section have the ability to affect a client's activity and participation as defined in the ICF model. For example, a person's hearing impairment will need to be considered when conducting assessments on an aging individual, but it will also influence domains of function that a recreational therapist might need to address to determine activity limitations and participation in important life domains such as learning and applying knowledge (d1); communication (d3); interpersonal interactions (d7); and involvement in community, social, and civic life (d9). Being aware of aging-specific issues that might affect older clients in recreational therapy programs is important, and understanding how these factors may be related to the ICF will improve the recreational therapist's ability to clearly communicate the client's needs and abilities to the treatment team after conducting assessments of their performance in different domains.

Age-Related Considerations When Assessing Older Adults

In addition to the factors noted previously, there are other challenges when assessing older adults. This is because age-related differences in the expression of some symptoms have been identified, but also due to the fact that some changes they experience are incorrectly attributed to age. In this section, two common age-related considerations when assessing older adults will be discussed: the assessment of depression and distinguishing between dementia and delirium.

Assessing Depression

One common myth is that depression is a normal part of aging; this is not true. That said, older adults are at an increased risk for experiencing depression due to the prevalence of chronic conditions and other changes they experience during this life stage (CDC, 2017). For example, hearing loss is independently associated with the development of depression (Chang-Quan, Bi-Rong, Lu, Yue, & Liu, 2010) as well as loneliness and social isolation (Pronk, Deeg, Smits, van Tilburg, Kuik, Festen, et al., 2011), which could lead to depressive symptoms. The rate of major depression in older adults is estimated to range from less than 1 percent to 5 percent of adults who reside in the community, 11.5 percent to 13.5 percent of those who are in the hospital or require home health care respectively, and up to 50 percent of older adults in long-term care facilities (CDC, 2017; Hoover, Siegle, Lucas, Kalay, Gabota, Devanand, et al., 2010). However, it is widely acknowledged that depression among older adults is seriously undetected, undiagnosed, and undertreated, particularly in primary care settings (Allan, Valkanova, & Ebmeier, 2014).

One of the reasons why depression is overlooked with the aging population is because many of the symptoms coincide with other problems encountered by older adults. Some of the characteristics of depression in this age group include memory problems (b144), confusion (b114), social withdrawal (d9205), inability to sleep (b134), vague complaints of pain (b280), change in appetite (b1302), irritability (b126), and weight loss (b530) (National Alliance on Mental Illness, 2009). In addition, some older adults do not identify sadness as their main symptom, and instead note less obvious symptoms of depression or may be less willing to talk about their feelings (National Institute of Mental Health, n.d.). Because older adults may have atypical presentations of depression when compared to younger populations, this may make the assessment of depression more difficult. This is complicated by the fact that many of the scales available to assess depression were not originally designed for older adults and lack proper validation for use with this population (Holroyd & Clayton, 2000). Thus, it is important to use a depression scale specific to the aging population when assessing depression with older adults. Many depression scales are appropriate for use by a CTRS (e.g., Geriatric Depression Scale); however, depending on the measure chosen, the assessment might need to be completed by an individual with counseling or psychiatric credentials. If this is the case, recreational therapists might consider collaborating with one of the mental health professionals in their facility to conduct this assessment.

Differentiating Between Delirium and Dementia

Another myth about aging is that confusion and dementia are not unusual. While there are some age-related changes in cognition that occur, significant confusion among older adults is not expected or normal. Two potential causes of such confusion in older adults are delirium and dementia. Delirium is as an acute state in which symptoms emerge over a period of days or weeks and fluctuate over a 24-hour period; it is often under-recognized in the aging population. It is present in approximately 10 to 30 percent of hospitalized elderly patients (Gagliardi, 2008) and in up to 60 percent of patients in nursing homes or post-acute care settings (Kiely, Bergmann, Jones, Murphy, Orav, & Marcantonio, 2004); however, it is reversible. A hallmark characteristic of delirium is the presence of an underlying medical disorder, and possible causes of delirium in the aging population include metabolic disorders, infections, toxins, or severe sleep deprivation. Patients with delirium may have lethargy, difficulty focusing, disorganized thinking, altered levels of consciousness, memory deficits, emotional disturbances (e.g., paranoia, apathy), or even psychomotor disturbances such as hallucinations (Inouye, 2006). Once the underlying cause of delirium is treated, the adult's confusion should abate.

Dementia is defined as a chronic state with a slow and gradual onset due to a chronic disorder such as Alzheimer's disease or Parkinson's disease that progressively worsens over time. Typically, dementia has no effect on an individual's level of consciousness or attention until the late stages, although loss of memory for recent events is especially evident (Alzheimer's Association, 2017).

While dementia and delirium are two independent diagnoses, they frequently coexist. In fact, dementia is a leading risk factor for delirium, and there is an increased incidence of new cognitive decline and dementia after delirium (Fong, Inouye, & Jones, 2017). Recreational therapists need to be aware of the disturbances in clients' attention (b140), because this is a key distinguishing factor between delirium and dementia. The ICF code for delirium related to global mental function is b110 (consciousness functions), while dementia is specifically noted under b117 (intellectual functions). A misdiagnosis or attribution of cognitive impairment during assessment to dementia may further delay treatment for the underlying medical disorder that is causing the delirium.

Considerations When Working With Adults With Dementia

As discussed in the previous sections, some of the changes that occur with aging make the assessment process slightly more complicated when working with older adults. This is particularly true when working with individuals who have dementia. Dementia impairs an individual's ability to clearly communicate as well as their ability to understand and process information. Thus, the responsibility lies with the therapist or clinician to promote effective communication during the assessment process.

Persons with dementia frequently communicate information through their behaviors. Thus, many nonverbal behaviors that individuals exhibit (e.g., agitation, restlessness, aggression, combativeness) are often an expression of the individuals' unmet needs (e.g., pain, hunger, thirst) (Zembrzuski, 2013). It is important to try to interpret the underlying meaning of these behaviors when they are demonstrated by patients and not just dismiss them as symptoms of the dementia. For example, there is evidence that pain is underdetected and poorly managed in adults with dementia in long-term and acute care (Lichtner, Dowding, Esterhuizen, Closs, Long, Corbet, et al., 2014). However, observational tools have been developed to assess the presence of pain in adults with mild to moderate dementia based on the interpretation of behavioral cues such as facial expressions, negative vocalization, body language, changes in activity patterns, and changes in interpersonal interactions (American Geriatrics Society, 2002). Research has suggested that these objective assessments are reliable and valid (Jordan, Regnard, O'Brien, & Hughes, 2012).

Individuals with dementia may be able to answer simple and direct questions when they require only a "yes" or "no" response. They may also be able to make choices among options when the options are limited; using too many options will likely cause confusion and frustration for the individual. When possible, try to formulate the questions of your assessment in such a way that you are able to include the individual in the assessment process.

CASE STUDY

Determining Areas of Needed Assessment

Yesterday an 80-year-old female, Lucy, was admitted to an acute care facility by her family after they found her disoriented with signs of memory loss and apathy. Her son was unsure how long she had been exhibiting these behaviors but was afraid to let her continue living in her home alone. He told the medical staff upon their arrival at the facility that his mother also has some hearing deficits. Jennifer is the recreational therapist in this facility and needs to conduct her initial assessment with the new patient. Based on the information in this chapter, what are some of the things that Jennifer needs to consider as she interviews Lucy?

First, given that Lucy is hard of hearing it would be important for Jennifer to conduct the assessment in a quiet location where there are few distractions. Next, since her family is unsure of how long Lucy has had this cognitive impairment, Jennifer might want to check whether other staff already assessed her attention and ability to focus, because this could provide some insight into whether Lucy may be experiencing delirium, dementia, or perhaps both. Memory loss and confusion may also be indicators of depression in older adults. Thus, this would also be important information that Jennifer should review or collect during the assessment process so that the treatment team could best address Lucy's health concerns and needs. Given Lucy's cognitive state, some of the tips for assessing clients with dementia might also prove useful as Jennifer speaks with her. This includes using simple and direct questions, providing limited choices, paying attention to any nonverbal behaviors that she might exhibit during the assessment process, and consulting family members for additional information. Finally, when Jennifer is determining the leisure interests and hobbies of this new patient she needs to be cognizant of her own stereotypes about older adults and make sure she does not have preconceived ideas of Lucy's preferred activities and interests, because this information will influence the choice of interventions used in recreational therapy during her hospitalization.

Family members and caregivers are a good source of information needed in recreational therapy assessments as well, but the therapist should make a concerted effort to obtain information from the patient's perspective since this may not align directly with information that is provided by others. It is also important to remember that dementia affects the adults' cognitive abilities, not their physical functioning. Thus, many older adults with dementia are quite capable of performing assessments of physical abilities such as gait and balance. In these situations, the therapist might find it useful to use gestures or model the desired behavior to increase the individual's understanding of what is being asked.

Finding Assessments to Use With Older Adults

Searching for assessments that are appropriate for use with older adults can be done quickly. There are a number of free and publicly available resources to find appropriate assessments for use with this population. In this section, we'll review the Rehabilitation Measures Database, a website that can help the recreational therapist find assessments by area of concern, as well as the Dementia Practice Guidelines for Treatment of Disturbing Behaviors and the Buettner Assessment of Needs, Diagnoses and Interests for Recreational Therapy (Buettner, Connolly, & Richeson, 2011).

Rehabilitation Measures Database

The Rehabilitation Measures Database (Rehabmeasures.org) is a website developed by the Rehabilitation Institute of Chicago (RIC) and the Center for Rehabilitation Outcomes Research (CROR). The tagline for the website is "The Rehabilitation Clinician's Place to Find the Best Instruments to Screen Patients and Monitor Their Progress." From the website, a recreational therapist can choose from a wide range of areas of assessment (ranging from activities of daily living to vision) or search

by diagnosis, length of test, or cost. Once an area is chosen to search, the website provides a summary of the assessment, including the length of time and training required to administer the test, cost, and populations that have been tested with the assessment. A detailed instrument review is provided, as is a link to the instrument. Notably, each instrument review includes which ICF domains the assessment covers! It is impossible to review most of the assessments found in the Rehabilitation Measures Database that are appropriate for older adults, but a sample discussion of assessments from the Participation, Mood, and Quality of Life categories are provided here. Please note that there are many more assessments available on the website that may meet the population or clinician's needs.

Participation

The Life Satisfaction Questionnaire 9 (LiSAT-9) assesses a variety of areas of life satisfaction, including (but not limited to) sex life (d7702), leisure situations (d920), family life (d6 and d9), and social contacts (d998) (Anke & Fugl-Meyer, 2003). This nine-item questionnaire does not have limits on who can administer it, and it is free to obtain. The LiSAT-9 has been found to be valid and reliable in the following populations: stroke, traumatic brain injury, multiple sclerosis, spinal cord injury, trauma, and chronic pain (c.f. Anke & Fugl-Meyer, 2003; Boonstra, Reneman, Posthumus, Stewart, & Schiphorst Preuper, 2008; Post, van Leeuwen, van Koppenhagen, & de Groot, 2012).

The Physical Activity Scale for the Elderly (PASE) evaluates the amount of self-reported physical activity an older adult engages in during occupational, household, and leisure activities in the previous seven-day period (d570, d920) (Washburn, McAuley, Katula, Mihalko, & Boileau, 1999; Washburn, Smith, Jette, & Janney, 1993). This 12-item questionnaire does not require training to administer, but it does have a fee of $125 for the administration and scoring manual. The PASE has been found to be reliable and valid in many older adult populations, including community-dwelling elders and individuals with hip osteoarthritis, cancer, knee pain, and joint replacement (c.f. Casartelli, Bolszak, Impellizzeri, & Maffiuletti, 2015; Cavanaugh & Crawford, 2014; Dinger, Oman, Taylor, Vesely, & Able, 2004).

Mood

The Patient Health Questionnaire (PHQ-9) is a nine-item questionnaire that takes one to three minutes to administer to determine the presence and intensity of depressive symptoms (Kroenke, Spitzer, & Williams, 2001). Mood is coded as b1263 (mental functions, psychic stability), and depression would be identified as impairments in mental functions, as well as potentially named as a health condition. The PHQ-9 is widely used and has been found to be valid and reliable in the following populations: cardiology, dementia, general medical outpatients, oncology, Parkinson's disease, primary care, spinal cord injury, stroke, and traumatic brain injury (c.f. Gilbody, Richards, Brealey, & Hewitt, 2007; Hancock & Larner, 2009; Janneke, Hafsteinsdóttir, Lindeman, Burger, Grobbee, & Schuurmans, 2012; Klaiberg & Braehler, 2006; Krause, Saunders, Reed, Coker, Zhai, & Johnson, 2009).

Quality of Life

The World Health Organization Quality of Life-BREF (WHOQOL-BREF) takes approximately 10 to 15 minutes to administer, is free, and has been validated with community-dwelling older adults, older adults with a fear of falling, and older adults with depression, as well as transplant patients, wheelchair users, and those with diabetes, dementia, HIV, neurological illness, Parkinson's disease, spinal cord injury, stroke, or traumatic brain injury (c.f. Kuyken, Orley, Hudelson, & Sartorius, 1995; Lucas-Carrasco, Skevington, Gómez-Benito, Rejas, & March, 2011; World Health Organization, 1996). To be qualified to administer the WHOQOL-BREF, the clinician must read the manual. The self-report questionnaire assesses four domains of quality of life, including physical health (d570, d5702), psychological health (b122), environment (e1, e2, e3, e4, e5), and social relationships (d998), and includes 26 items.

Dementia Practice Guidelines for Recreation Therapists: Treatment of Disturbing Behaviors

The Dementia Practice Guidelines (DPG) for Recreation Therapists is designed to provide evidence-based treatment guidelines, describe relevant models and theories, and discuss the literature and indications for recreational therapy practice for working with individuals with dementia who have disruptive behaviors (Buettner & Fitzsimmons, 2008). In the section that focuses specifically on the recreational therapy treatment process for treating disturbing behaviors, a behavior flow record is available to chart when the behavior occurs, the interventions that have been attempted, and the resulting change (or lack thereof) in behavior. This checklist could be very helpful in monitoring progress and modifying disturbing behaviors.

The DPG also provides a brief description of seven screening tools that may be used to determine the baseline aptitude of individuals with dementia. In screening for cognition, the DPG describes the Global Deterioration Scale and the Mini-Mental State Exam. The Global Deterioration Scale (GDS; Reisberg, Ferris, de Leon, & Crook, 1982) is a measure that helps caregivers determine where their loved one is in the spectrum of Alzheimer's disease (b114). The GDS identifies seven different stages; stages 1 to 4 are identified as the stages prior to dementia, and stages 5 to 7 indicate that the individual needs assistance in their daily life. Another cognitive screening tool mentioned is the Mini-Mental State Exam (MMSE) (b114). The DPG describes the 30-item measure (Folstein, Folstein, & McHugh, 1975), but there is now also a six item version of the MMSE (Callahan, Unverzagt, Hui, Perkins, & Hendrie, 2002). The six-item version is publicly available online (www.public-health.uiowa.edu/icmha/outreach/documents/SIXITE1.PDF), whereas the 30-item version requires a fee. The six-item MMSE also has demonstrated strong reliability and validity.

It is important to note that the Montreal Cognitive Assessment (MoCA) is becoming increasingly preferred to the MMSE when working with older adults, because it is more sensitive to finding mild cognitive impairment (MCI); in fact, a recent study found that the MMSE detected 18 percent of MCI, while the MoCA detected 90 percent of MCI (Nasreddine, Phillips, Bédirian, Charbonneau, Whitehead, Collin, et al., 2005). The MoCA takes approximately 10 minutes to administer and is publicly available.

In terms of evaluating client outcomes, the DPG recommends six standard measures that cover agitation (b1268), apathy (b1264), aggression (b126), two scales of depression (b1263), and wandering (b114) and includes a copy of each of these measures in the appendixes. These measures are briefly described below.

- For agitation, the DPG recommends the Cohen-Mansfield Agitation Inventory (CMAI) (b1268) (Cohen-Mansfield, 1986). This scale measures 29 behaviors that indicate agitation and has adequate reliability.
- The Apathy Evaluation Scale (AES) is based on the observation of the caregiver and evaluates neurological-based apathy (b1264) in individuals with cognitive impairment. The AES includes 18 items and has correlations with loss of motivation (Marin, 1996).
- The Overt Aggression Scale (OAS) evaluates aggression in four categories: verbal, physical against self, physical against others, and physical against objects (b126). Seven items evaluate the frequency of these behaviors over the past week (Yudofsky, Silver, Jackson, Endicott, & Williams, 1986).
- The Geriatric Depression Scale (GDS) identifies the presence of depressive symptoms (b1263) in older adults. A 15-item or 30-item GDS is available for use, both demonstrating strong validity and reliability (Yesavage, Brink, Rose, Lum, Huang, Adey, et al., 1983).

- The Cornell Scale for Depression (Alexopoulos, Abrams, Young, & Shamoian, 1988) has 19 items and uses information from both the individual and a staff member perspective to evaluate depressive symptoms (b1263), making this scale appropriate for use with individuals with impaired cognition.
- The Algase Wandering Scale (AWS) has 28 items that evaluate five dimensions of wandering (b114). This scale has demonstrated adequate reliability and validity (Algase, Beattie, Bogue, & Yao, 2001).

Buettner Assessment of Needs, Diagnoses and Interests for Recreation Therapy

A specific assessment for recreational therapy in long-term care facilities is the Buettner Assessment of Needs, Diagnoses and Interests for Recreation Therapy (BANDI-RT; Buettner, Connolly, & Richeson, 2011). This assessment is free and publicly available. BANDI-RT aligns with the Minimum Data Set 3.0 (MDS 3.0), a standardized assessment tool that is used in long-term care facilities to document information about residents. The BANDI-RT collects general information about the resident, such as language (b16700, d3150, d330), past occupation (d850), and family members (e315). It also takes into account special considerations relevant to the provision of recreation therapy services, such as fall risk (d450), presence of one-sided weakness (b730), needing assist to ambulate (d450), swallowing difficulties (b735), dietary restriction (d550), types of medication, and health conditions including recent fractures, seizures, allergies, or diabetes; and mental status information, such as cognition, delirium, or mood (b110-1149).

The BANDI-RT section on leisure history and interests (d920) asks about interests in the following areas: creative, entertainment, games, home activities, nature/outdoors, physical activities, social/community, technology, well-being, and new interests. The next section summarizes the functioning levels by having the recreational therapist explore the other areas of the MDS 3.0, including the following sections:

- B: Sensory (b2)
- C: Cognitive (b1)
- D: Psychosocial/mood (b122)
- E: Behavioral (b126)
- F: Personal preferences
- G: Physical/mobility (d4)
- H: Continence (d530)
- I: Active disease (health condition)
- J: Pain (health condition)
- M: Skin (b8)

Subsequently, the BANDI-RT has a section for treatment considerations that include behavioral issues (b122), communication (d3), family/friends (e3), functional (b7), physical (b7), psychiatric/emotional (b1-199), sensory (b2), social (e3), and spiritual considerations (d930). The final section of the BANDI-RT identifies potential interventions, includes an area to document the physician order, and has space for treatment planning. The BANDI-RT is a holistic and comprehensive assessment tool that can assist the recreational therapist in mainstreaming treatment planning with the treatment team. The BANDI-RT has demonstrated strong content validity and test-retest reliability (Buettner, Richeson, & Connolly, 2012).

CASE STUDY

Putting the Pieces Together

Ms. Carol Ramirez is a new resident in a long-term care facility based in Tucson, Arizona. One of the recreational therapists at the facility, Curt Swinney, is assigned to do her intake evaluation. The first thing Curt does is review her chart to learn about her history and her background. He finds that she is 75 years old, she has been widowed for two years, and in the years since her husband's death, she has become increasingly confused, demonstrating poor short-term memory but adequate long-term memory. Her thoughts appear more disorganized, her speech is tangential, and her family physician is the one who has recommended that she move into a long-term care facility. She does not have children, but she has a lot of support from friends and family. After reviewing the chart, Curt fills in as much information as he can on the BANDI-RT. He then meets with Ms. Ramirez to fill out the other sections. They meet in the lounge, a noisy room that has TVs on at a loud volume and where many residents are socializing. On this particular day, bingo is being played in the room, so there are frequent distractions and loud shouts from participants. Curt finds Ms. Ramirez easy to converse with but the information she provides him from section to section is unreliable and contradictory. Ms. Ramirez indicates that her primary leisure interests have been physical and social in nature; however, when he suggests that they go for a walk together, she refuses, saying, "I hate to walk." He suggests that they go to exercise group, but she states, "I hate to exercise." She then starts to act aggressively toward him.

Questions for Consideration

1. Curt shares Ms. Ramirez's reaction with an attending physician. The physician states, "Well, of course she is confused. She is 75 years old." How should Curt respond?

2. Describe the differences between delirium and dementia. Which do you think Ms. Ramirez is experiencing? What is your rationale for that choice?

3. In addition to the BANDI-RT, is there another assessment mentioned in this chapter that Curt should include? If yes, which one, and why?

Summary

Assessing older adults is an important part of recreational therapy practice. In this chapter, we reviewed important considerations for the RT professional who is working with older adults. We also identified a number of appropriate, reliable, and valid assessments for use with this population. Providing age-appropriate assessment and care is essential in RT practice, and therapists are encouraged to implement these practices with their client population.

REFLECTION QUESTIONS

1. What groups may have stereotypes about aging, and how can these affect the assessment process?

2. What are some health-related or clinical setting factors that might interfere with the assessment process of aging individuals? How do they relate to areas of the ICF?

3. What are some reasons that depression is often overlooked and undiagnosed in older adults?

4. What are some similarities and differences in the signs and symptoms of dementia and delirium in older adults?

5. What are some factors that recreational therapists need to consider when assessing individuals with dementia?

6. What are some factors that recreational therapists need to consider when choosing an assessment for older adults?

7. What assessments might be appropriate for recreational therapists to use when measuring the (a) physical, (b) cognitive, (c) emotional, and (d) social functioning of older adults? What areas of the ICF do these assessments address?

REFERENCES

Alexopoulos, G.S., Abrams, R.C., Young, R.C., & Shamoian, C.A. (1988). Cornell scale for depression in dementia. *Biological Psychiatry, 23*(3), 271-284.

Algase, D.L., Beattie, E.R., Bogue, E.L., & Yao, L. (2001). The Algase wandering scale: Initial psychometrics of a new caregiver reporting tool. *American Journal of Alzheimer's Disease & Other Dementias, 16*(3), 141-152.

Allan, C.E., Valkanova, V., & Ebmeier, K.P. (2014). Depression in older people is underdiagnosed. *Practitioner, 258*(1771), 19-22.

Alzheimer's Association. (2017). Delirium or dementia: Do you know the difference? Retrieved May 17, 2017, from www.alz.org/norcal/in_my_community_17590.asp

American Geriatrics Society. (2002). Panel on persistent pain in older persons: The management of persistent pain in older persons. *Journal of the American Geriatrics Society, 50*, S205-S224.

Anke, A.G.W., & Fugl-Meyer, A.R. (2003). Life satisfaction several years after severe multiple trauma—a retrospective investigation. *Clinical Rehabilitation, 17*(4), 431-442.

Boonstra, A.M., Reneman, M.F., Posthumus, J.B., Stewart, R.E., & Schiphorst Preuper, H.R. (2008). Reliability of the life satisfaction questionnaire to assess patients with chronic musculoskeletal pain. *International Journal of Rehabilitation Research, 31*(2), 181-183.

Buettner, L., Connolly, P., & Richeson, N. (2011). Buettner assessment of needs, diagnoses and interests for recreation therapy in LTC (BANDI-RT). Retrieved from https://usm.maine.edu/rls/bandi-rt

Buettner, L., & Fitzsimmons, S. (2008). *Dementia practice guidelines for recreational therapists: Treatment of disturbing behaviors.* Hattiesburg, MS: American Therapeutic Recreation Association.

Buettner, L.L., Richeson, N., Connolly, P. (2012). Content validity, reliability, and treatment outcomes of the

Buettner assessment of needs, diagnoses and interests for recreational therapy in long-term care (BANDI-RT). *American Journal of Recreation Therapy, 11*(1).

Callahan, C.M., Unverzagt, F.W., Hui, S.L., Perkins, A.J., & Hendrie, H.C. (2002). Six-item screener to identify cognitive impairment among potential subjects for clinical research. *Medical Care, 40*(9), 771-781.

Carroll, L.J., Cassidy, J.D., Cancelliere, C., Côté, P., Hincapié, C.A., Kristman, V.L., et al. (2014). Systematic review of the prognosis after mild traumatic brain injury in adults: Cognitive, psychiatric, and mortality outcomes: Results of the International Collaboration on Mild Traumatic Brain Injury Prognosis. *Archives of Physical Medicine and Rehabilitation, 95*(3 Suppl 2), S152-173.

Casartelli, N.C., Bolszak, S., Impellizzeri, F.M., & Maffiuletti, N.A. (2015). Reproducibility and validity of the physical activity scale for the elderly (PASE) questionnaire in patients after total hip arthroplasty. *Physical Therapy, 95*(1), 86-94.

Cavanaugh, J.T., & Crawford, K. (2014). Life-space assessment and physical activity scale for the elderly: Validity of proxy informant responses. *Archives of Physical Medicine and Rehabilitation, 95*(8), 1527-1532.

Centers for Disease Control and Prevention (CDC). (2017). Depression is not a normal part of growing older. Retrieved May 17, 2017, from www.cdc.gov/aging/mentalhealth/depression.htm

Chang-Quan, H., Bi-Rong, D., Lu, Z.C., Yue, J.R., & Liu, Q.X. (2010). Chronic diseases and risk for depression in old age: A meta-analysis of published literature. *Ageing Research Review, 9*(2), 131-141.

Cohen-Mansfield, J. (1986). Agitated behaviors in the elderly: II. Preliminary results in the cognitively deteriorated. *Journal of the American Geriatrics Society, 34*(10), 722-727.

Dinger, M.K., Oman, R.F., Taylor, E.L., Vesely, S.K., & Able, J. (2004). Stability and convergent validity of the physical activity scale for the elderly (PASE). *Journal of Sports Medicine and Physical Fitness, 44*(2), 186-192.

Figueroa, J.J., Basford, J.R., & Low, P.A. (2010). Preventing and treating orthostatic hypotension: As easy as A, B, C. *Cleveland Clinic Journal of Medicine, 77*(5), 298-306. doi:10.3949/ccjm.77a.0911

Folstein, M.F., Folstein, S.E., & McHugh, P.R. (1975). Mini-mental state: A practical method for grading the cognitive state of patients for the clinician. *Journal of Psychiatry Research, 12,* 189-198.

Fong, T.G., Inouye, S.K., & Jones, R.N. (2017). Delirium, dementia, and decline. *JAMA Psychiatry, 74*(3), 212-213. doi:10.1001/jamapsychiatry.2016.3812

Gagliardi, J.P. (2008). Differentiating between depression, delirium, and dementia in elderly patients. *Virtual Mentor, 10*(6), 383-388. Retrieved from http://journalofethics.ama-assn.org/2008/06/pdf/cprl1-0806.pdf

Gilbody, S., Richards, D., Brealey, S., & Hewitt, C. (2007). Screening for depression in medical settings with the patient health questionnaire (PHQ): A diagnostic meta-analysis. *Journal of General Internal Medicine, 22*(11), 1596-1602.

Hancock, P., & Larner, A. (2009). Clinical utility of Patient Health Questionnaire-9 (PHQ-9) in memory clinics. *International Journal of Psychiatry in Clinical Practice, 13*(3), 188-191.

Higashi, R.T., Tillack, A.A., Steinman, M., Harper, M., & Johnson, C.B. (2012). Elder care as "frustrating" and "boring": Understanding the persistence of negative attitudes toward older patients among physicians-in-training. *Journal of Aging Studies, 26,* 476-483. doi: 10.1016/j.jaging.2012.06.007

Holroyd, S., & Clayton, A.H. (2000). Measuring depression in the elderly: Which scale is best. *Medscape General Medicine, 2*(4). http://www.medscape.com/viewarticle/430554

Hoover, D.R., Siegel, M., Lucas, J., Kalay, E., Gabota, D., Devanand, D.P., et al. (2010). Depression in the first year of stay for elderly long-term nursing home residents in the U.S.A. *International Psychogeriatrics,* 1-11.

Inouye, S.K. (2006). Delirum in older persons. *New England Journal of Medicine, 354,* 1157-1165. doi: 10.1056/NEJMra052321

Janneke, M., Hafsteinsdóttir, T., Lindeman, E., Burger, H., Grobbee, D., & Schuurmans, M. (2012). An efficient way to detect poststroke depression by subsequent administration of a 9-item and a 2-item patient health questionnaire. *Stroke, 43*(3), 854-856.

Jordan, A., Regnard, C., O'Brien, J.T., & Hughes, J.C. (2012). Pain and distress in advanced dementia: Choosing the right tools for the job. *Palliative Medicine, 26,* 873-878. doi:10.1177/0269216311412227

Kiely, D.K., Bergmann, M.A., Jones, R.N., Murphy, K.M., Orav, E.J., & Marcantonio, E.R. (2004). Characteristics associated with delirium persistence among newly admitted post-acute facility patients. *Journals of Gerontology: Biological and Medical Sciences, 59,* 344-349.

Klaiberg, A., & Braehler, E. (2006). Validity of the brief patient health questionnaire mood scale (PHQ-9) in the general population. *General Hospital Psychiatry, 28,* 71-77.

Krause, J.S., Saunders, L.L., Reed, K.S., Coker, J., Zhai, Y., & Johnson, E. (2009). Comparison of the patient health questionnaire and the older adult health and mood questionnaire for self-reported depressive symptoms after spinal cord injury. *Rehabilitation Psychology, 54*(4), 440-448.

Kroenke, K., Spitzer, R., & Williams, J.B. (2001). The PHQ-9: Validity of a brief depression symptom severity measure. *Journal of General Internal Medicine, 16*(9), 606-613.

Kuyken, W., Orley, J., Hudelson, P., & Sartorius, N. (1995). The World Health Organization quality of life assessment (WHOQOL): Position paper from the World Health Organization. *Social Science in Medicine, 41*(10), 1403-1409.

Lamont, R.A., Swift, H.J., & Abrams, D. (2015). A review and meta-analysis of age-based stereotype threat: Negative stereotypes, not facts, do the damage. *Psychology and Aging, 30*(1), 180-193. Retrieved from http://dx.doi.org/10.1037/a0038586

Lichtner, V., Dowding, D., Esterhuizen, P., Closs, S.J., Long, A.F., Corbet, A., & Briggs, M. (2014). Pain assessment for people with dementia: A systematic review of systematic reviews of pain assessment tools. *BMC Geriatrics, 14*, 138. Retrieved from www.biomedcentral.com/1471-2318/14/138

Lin, F.R. (2011). Hearing loss and cognition among older adults in the United States. *Journal of Gerontology: Biological and Medical Sciences, 66*(10), 1131-1136. PubMed: 21768501

Lipsitz, L.A. (2017). Orthostatic hypotension and falls. *Journal of the American Geriatrics Society, 65*, 270-271. doi:10.1111/jgs.14745

Lucas-Carrasco, R., Skevington, S.M., Gómez-Benito, J., Rejas, J., & March, J. (2011). Using the WHOQOL-BREF in persons with dementia: A validation study. *Alzheimer Disease and Associated Disorders, 25*(4), 345-351.

Marin, R.S. (1996). Apathy: Concept, syndrome, neural mechanisms, and treatment. *Seminars in Clinical Neuropsychiatry, 1*(4), 304-314.

McDowd, J., Filion, D., Pohl, P., Richards, L., & Stiers, W. (2003). Attentional abilities and functional outcomes following stroke. *Journals of Gerontology: Psychological and Social Science, 58*, P45-53.

McKenzie, E.L., & Brown, P.M. (2014). Nursing students' intentions to work in dementia care: Influence of age, ageism, and perceived barriers. *Educational Gerontology, 40*, 618-633.

Murray, M.D., & Callahan, C.M. (2003). Improving medication use for older adults: An integrated research agenda. *Annals of Internal Medicine, 139*(5), 425-429.

Nasreddine, Z.S., Phillips, N.A., Bédirian, V., Charbonneau, S., Whitehead, V., Collin, I., & Chertkow, H. (2005). The Montreal cognitive assessment, MoCA: A brief screening tool for mild cognitive impairment. *Journal of the American Geriatrics Society, 53*(4), 695-699.

National Alliance on Mental Illness. (2009). Depression in older persons. Retrieved May 17, 2017, from www.ncoa.org/wp-content/uploads/Depression_Older_Persons_FactSheet_2009.pdf

National Institute of Mental Health. (n.d.). Older adults and depression. Retrieved on May 17, 2017, from www.nimh.nih.gov/health/publications/older-adults-and-depression/qf-16-7697_153371.pdf

National Institute on Deafness and Other Communication Disorders (NIDCD). (2016). Quick statistics about hearing. U.S. Department of Health and Human Services, National Institutes of Health. Retrieved April 10, 2017, from www.nidcd.nih.gov/health/statistics/quick-statistics-hearing

Post, M.W., van Leeuwen, C.M., van Koppenhagen, C.F., & de Groot, S. (2012). Validity of the life satisfaction questions, the life satisfaction questionnaire, and the satisfaction with life scale in persons with spinal cord injury. *Archives of Physical Medicine and Rehabilitation, 93*(10), 1832-1837.

Pronk, M., Deeg, D.J., Smits, C., van Tilburg, T.G., Kuik, D.J., Festen, J.M., & Kramer, S.E. (2011). Prospective effects of hearing status on loneliness and depression in older persons: Identification of subgroups. *International Journal of Audiology, 50*(12), 887-896. http://dx.doi.org/10.3109/14992027.2011.599871

Reisberg, B., Ferris, S.H., de Leon, M.J., & Crook, T. (1982). The global deterioration scale for assessment of primary degenerative dementia. *The American Journal of Psychiatry, 139*, 1136-1139.

Rubenstein, L.Z. (2006). Falls in older people: Epidemiology, risk factors, and strategies for prevention. *Age & Ageing, 35-S2*, ii37-ii41.

Washburn, R.A., McAuley, E., Katula, J., Mihalko, S.L., & Boileau, R.A. (1999). The physical activity scale for the elderly (PASE): Evidence for validity. *Journal of Clinical Epidemiology, 52*(7), 643-651.

Washburn, R.A., Smith, K.W., Jette, A.M., & Janney, C.A. (1993). The physical activity scale for the elderly (PASE): Development and evaluation. *Journal of Clinical Epidemiology, 46*(2), 153-162.

Weeks, J.C., & Hasher, L. (2014). The disruptive—and beneficial—effects of distraction on older adults' cognitive performance. *Frontiers in Psychology, 5*, 133. doi:10.3389/fpsyg.2014.00133

Weiss, A., Grossman, E., Beloosesky, Y., & Grinblat, J. (2002). Orthostatic hypotension in acute geriatric ward: Is it a consistent finding? *Archives of Internal Medicine, 162*, 2369-2374.

Wilson, I.R., Schoen, C., Neuman, P., Strollo, M.K., Rogers, W.H., Chang, H., et al. (2007). Physician-patient communication about prescription medication nonadherence: A 50-state study of America's seniors. *Journal of General Internal Medicine, Jan 22*(1), 6-12.

World Health Organization. (1996). WHOQOL-BREF: Introduction, administration, scoring and generic version of the assessment: Field trial version, December 1996.

World Health Organization. (2001). *International classification of functioning, disability and health.* Geneva: Author.

Yesavage, J.A., Brink, T.L., Rose, T.L., Lum, O., Huang, V., Adey, M., & Leirer, V.O. (1983). Development and validation of a geriatric depression screening scale: A preliminary report. *Journal of Psychiatric Research, 17*(1), 37-49.

Yudofsky, S.C., Silver, J.M., Jackson, W., Endicott, J., & Williams, D. (1986). The overt aggression scale for the objective rating of verbal and physical aggression. *The American Journal of Psychiatry, 143*(1), 35-39.

Yueh, B., Shapiro, N., MacLean, C.H., & Shekelle, P.G. (2003). Screening and management of adult hearing loss in primary care: Scientific review. *JAMA, 289*(15), 1976-1985.

Zembrzuski, C. (2013). Communication difficulties: Assessment and interventions in hospitalized older adults with dementia. *Best Practices in Nursing Care to Older Adults with Dementia*, D7. Alzheimer's Association. Retrieved May 12, 2017, from https://consultgeri.org/try-this/dementia/issue-d7.pdf

ADDITIONAL RESOURCES

Brink, T.L., Yesavage, J.A., Lum, O., Heersema, P., Adey, M.B., & Rose, T.L. (1982). Screening tests for geriatric depression. *Clinical Gerontologist, 1*, 37-44.

Gill, T.M., Williams, C.S., & Tinetti, M.E. (1995). Assessing risk for the onset of functional dependence among older adults: The role of physical performance. *Journal of the American Geriatrics Society, 43*(6), 603-609.

Huang, H.C., Gau, M.L., Lin, W.C., & George, K. (2003). Assessing risk of falling in older adults. *Public Health Nursing, 20*(5), 399-411.

Kane, R.L, & Kane, R.A. (2000). *Assessing older persons: Measures, meaning, and practical applications.* Oxford, UK: Oxford University Press.

Logsdon, R.G., Gibbons, L.E., McCurry, S.M., & Teri, L. (2002). Assessing quality of life in older adults with cognitive impairment. *Psychosomatic Medicine, 64*(3), 510-519.

Marin, R.S., Biedrzycki, R.C., & Firinciogullari, S. (1991). Reliability and validity of the apathy evaluation scale. *Psychiatry Research, 38*(2), 143-162.

Rikli, R.E., & Jones, C.J. (1997). Assessing physical performance in independent older adults: Issues and guidelines. *Journal of Aging and Physical Activity, 5*(3), 244-261.

CHAPTER 6

Assessment and Behavioral Health

Bryan P. McCormick, PhD, CTRS

Gretchen Snethen, PhD, CTRS

LEARNING OBJECTIVES

Upon completion of the text, the student will demonstrate:

- Knowledge of transdiagnostic processes common to many major behavioral health disorders.
- Knowledge of WHO's *International Classification of Functioning, Disability and Health* (ICF) functional domains relevant to behavioral health practice.
- Knowledge of sources for evidence-based instruments for use in behavioral health practice.
- Knowledge of recreational therapy instruments identified for behavioral health practice.
- Skill in applying ICF functional domains to client assessment.

Although many definitions of assessment in RT focus on the *collection* of information as a basis for subsequent steps in service provision, others have emphasized the *interpretation* of collected information as the critical component in the assessment phase. We support the idea that, although the collection of relevant information as part of the assessment phase is critically important, it is the interpretation of these data that requires the clinical judgment and critical thinking of a trained recreational therapist (Austin & McCormick, 2013). Research on RT practice indicates that more than 80 percent of practicing recreational therapists report using an individualized assessment process, and this appears to be even higher in behavioral and mental health practice (Kemeny, Hutchins, & Cooke, 2016). Additionally, Hunsley and Mash (2007) noted that in order for assessment to be a solid foundation for evidence-based practice, assessment processes and tools have to be clinically relevant, culturally sensitive, and sci-entifically sound—that is, the assessment pro-cess itself should also be evidence based. This speaks to the need for the use of established practices and instruments in the assessment process. Almost 70 percent of practicing RT professionals in mental health settings report using a standardized assessment measure, which appears to be comparable to practice in developmental disabilities and pediatrics but is a lower percentage than physical medicine and rehabilitation (Kemeny et al., 2016).

Although the process of assessment has been widely addressed in the TR literature, the content of assessment procedures, specific to broad areas of practice such as behavioral health, has been rarely addressed. Part of the reason for a lack of consensus on the content of assessment processes may have been a reliance by authors on the use of domains of behavior and function to discuss areas of function appro-priate to assess. These domains are frequently characterized as *physical*, *cognitive*, *social*, and *emotional*; however, additional domains, such as leisure, have been proposed, while others, such as social/emotional, have been combined (Burlingame & Blaschko, 2010). While this typology has been used for almost a century in health care (Burlingame & Blaschko, 2010),

its lack of precision may present problems in identifying specific aspects of function to assess. A more precise approach to describ-ing aspects of functioning was developed by the World Health Organization in 2001 and presented in the *International Classification of Functioning, Disability and Health* (ICF; World Health Organization, 2001). This approach has been increasingly adopted across health care disciplines and provides a common terminol-ogy of function. Its use is seen increasingly in TR literature and textbooks (e.g., Porter, 2015b) and can provide a basis for identifying common areas of functional need across diverse behav-ioral and psychological disorders.

Transdiagnostic Perspective

In addition to the challenges of finding a common terminology to identify areas of func-tional need in behavioral health, the treatment of psychological disorders has also taken what has been characterized as a transdiagnostic approach in which specific diagnoses are of lesser importance while processes maintaining dysfunction across diagnoses are of greater focus (Barlow, 2011; Harvey, Watkins, Mansell, & Shafran, 2004; Kring & Sloan, 2010). For example, in major anxiety and depressive disorders there is selective attention paid to negative external stimuli, such that people only notice and act on negative self-referen-tial information. One of the strengths of this approach is that while many people may iden-tify a single, clearly defined psychological or behavioral disorder, single disorders are more frequently characterized as mild in severity, whereas those with multiple disorders are more frequently characterized as moderate to serious in severity (Kessler, Chiu, Demler, Merikangas, & Walters, 2005). Thus, those with moderate to serious severity are much more likely to be seen in treatment settings and presenting with multiple disorders. In addition, Harvey and colleagues (2004) asserted that comorbidities may reflect common vulnerabilities. For exam-ple, as much as 80 percent of people diagnosed with an eating disorder are also diagnosed with an anxiety disorder (Schwalberg, Barlow, Alger, & Howard, 1992).

A number of key processes have been identified that are implicated in the onset or maintenance of most major psychological disorders (Barlow, 2011; Harvey et al., 2004; Kring & Sloan, 2010). One process that cuts across many psychological disorders is emotional processing. For example, emotion and emotional regulation are implicated in over 75 percent of diagnostic categories in the *Diagnostic and Statistical Manual of Mental Disorders* (Werner & Gross, 2010). Additionally, attentional processes in which stimuli are selectively attended to are common in many major psychological disorders (Millan et al., 2012). This can be both when attentional processes are heightened, such as in post-traumatic stress disorder (PTSD), or weakened, as in attention deficit hyperactivity disorder (ADHD). In addition, memory processes are also implicated in multiple psychological disorders (Harvey et al., 2004). Again, memory can be implicated in terms of the selective retrieval of negative thoughts such as in social anxiety, as well as deficits in memory that can interfere with social functioning, as seen in schizophrenia.

Reasoning processes also cut across psychological diagnoses and may maintain dysfunction (Harvey et al., 2004). Reasoning involves such acts as interpreting stimuli, making attributions, and predicting future outcomes, as well as creating and testing hypotheses. An example of a reasoning process that may maintain dysfunction is the attributional bias seen in depression, in which those with depressive disorders often attribute failures to stable, global internal causes (e.g., "I'm no good": Seligman, 1991).

Thought processes are another area implicated in the onset and maintenance of many psychological and behavioral disorders (Harvey et al., 2004). These processes include such thought processes as intrusive thoughts, recurrent negative thinking, impaired metacognition, and reality monitoring. For example, adults with psychotic disorders may lack the metacognitive ability to synthesize and integrate experiences, making activities largely meaningless and potentially undermining motivation for any activity (Hasson-Ohayon, Arnon-Ribenfeld, Hamm, & Lysaker, 2017).

Finally, behavioral processes, including escape and avoidance behaviors as well as the development of dysfunctional safety seeking behaviors, such as compulsive hand washing, are seen across multiple diagnoses (Harvey et al., 2004). Additionally, behavioral activation and inhibition systems appear to be implicated across multiple disorders involving anxiety and mood dysfunction (Barlow, 2011; Brown & Barlow, 2009).

Part of the challenge in recreational therapy assessment in behavioral health settings is the degree to which our existing assessment instruments capture underlying processes maintaining dysfunction. There is reason to assume that RT assessment instruments have been relatively good at capturing behavioral processes because the profession has historically been focused on activities and patterns of recreation and leisure participation. Yet, the degree to which RT assessment instruments and processes focus on transdiagnostic processes is unexamined.

The *International Classification of Functioning, Disability and Health*

The *International Classification of Functioning, Disability and Health* (ICF) provides a tool for defining functional impairment and individual strengths within the areas of body function and structure, activities, and participation. The ICF does not contain specific diagnoses, which are known as *health conditions* in ICF terms. Instead, one must identify functional domains relevant to behavioral health practice. Those codes most relevant to behavioral health practice can be found in the areas of mental functions (b1), activities and participation (d), and environmental factors (e). However, the ICF Research Center has begun to identify ICF codes most relevant for certain health conditions, known as the *Core Sets*, and currently Core Sets exist for bipolar disorder, major depressive disorder, and schizophrenia spectrum disorder.

The transdiagnostic processes identified here align well with aspects of both specific mental functions as well as general tasks and demands as found in the ICF (see Transdiagnostic Processes and ICF Codes). The recreational therapy assessment process in behavioral health should be particularly attuned to functional needs in these areas.

Transdiagnostic Processes and ICF Codes

Attentional Processes

b140, Attention functions: "Specific mental functions of focusing on an external stimulus or internal experience for the required period of time. Inclusions: functions of sustaining attention, shifting attention, dividing attention, sharing attention; concentration; distractibility."

Memory Processes

b144, Memory functions: "Specific mental functions of registering and storing information and retrieving it as needed. Inclusions: functions of short-term and long-term memory, immediate, recent and remote memory; memory span; retrieval of memory; remembering; functions used in recalling and learning, such as in nominal, selective and dissociative amnesia."

Emotion Processes

b152, Emotional functions: "Specific mental functions related to the feeling and affective components of the processes of the mind. Inclusions: functions of appropriateness of emotion, regulation and range of emotion; affect; sadness, happiness, love, fear, anger, hate, tension, anxiety, joy, sorrow; lability of emotion; flattening of affect."

Reasoning Processes

b164, Higher-level cognitive functions: "Specific mental functions especially dependent on the frontal lobes of the brain, including complex goal-directed behaviors such as decision-making, abstract thinking, planning and carrying out plans, mental flexibility, and deciding which behaviors are appropriate under what circumstances; often called executive functions. Inclusions: functions of abstraction and organization of ideas; time management, insight and judgment; concept formation, categorization and cognitive flexibility."

Thought Processes

b160, Thought functions: "Specific mental functions related to the ideational component of the mind. Inclusions: functions of pace, form, control and content of thought; goal-directed thought functions, non-goal directed thought functions; logical thought functions, such as pressure of thought, flight of ideas, thought block, incoherence of thought, tangentiality, circumstantiality, delusions, obsessions and compulsions."

Behavioral Processes

d230, Carrying out daily routine: "Carrying out simple or complex and coordinated actions in order to plan, manage and complete the requirements of day-to-day procedures or duties, such as budgeting time and making plans for separate activities throughout the day. Inclusions: managing and completing the daily routine; managing one's own activity level."

d240, Handling stress and other psychological demands: "Carrying out simple or complex and coordinated actions to manage and control the psychological demands required to carry out tasks demanding significant responsibilities and involving stress, distraction, or crises, such as driving a vehicle during heavy traffic or taking care of many children. Inclusions: handling responsibilities; handling stress and crisis."

Source: World Health Organization. (2001). *International classification of health, disability and function*. Geneva: Author.

A review of RT assessment concerns related to specific diagnoses (Porter, 2015b) indicates that in addition to the core transdiagnostic domains, a number of other functional domains cut across many of the most commonly seen behavioral health diagnoses (table 6.1). Specifically, temperament and personality function (b126), energy and drive functions (b130) and experience of self and time (b180) are important areas to consider in the behavioral health assessment of mental functions. In addition, many major mental health conditions have other important areas of function to consider. Specifically, because many major mental health conditions have comorbidity with obesity (Becker, Margraf, Türke, Soeder, & Neumer, 2001), weight maintenance (b530) should likely be a common area to examine. Finally, although sexuality can be affected by mental health conditions (Zemishlany & Weizman, 2008), it is often overlooked within RT practice. While conversations about sexuality may be challenging, it is an important aspect of human function.

Beyond body function, there are also areas of activities and participation that are common across many major behavioral health diagnoses (table 6.2). One of the transdiagnostic processes that appears in all diagnoses is handling stress (d240), while managing daily routine (d230) appears as a functional area of need in many diagnoses. Another common area identified to assess is clients' looking after their own health needs (d570). The challenges posed by mental health conditions are frequently seen in the area of both basic interpersonal relationships (d710) and complex interpersonal relationships (d720), which have been identified as key areas to assess. Finally, function in recreation and leisure (d920) has been noted across almost all behavioral health conditions.

The final major chapter in the ICF considers environmental and personal factors in health and function (World Health Organization, 2001). These factors are frequently seen as elements of the physical, social, and personal environments that can be either barriers or facilitators to functioning. There appears to be less consensus or commonality in this area in terms of the functional domains to examine (table 6.3). It is worth noting that the mental health conditions for which there are Core Sets identified many more relevant functional domains in the environment chapter than many of the RT-specific sources (e.g., Neely, Parker, & Campbell, 2015; Porter, 2015a; Wood, Wyble, & Charters, 2015; Yang & Payne, 2015). Furthermore, there are several diagnoses that do not have environmental codes identified. One should not assume these areas do not influence the health and function of these individuals. Rather, these are areas for future research. Recreational therapists should consider these areas in order to better understand the factors that may promote or inhibit health and function.

In behavioral health, serious mental illnesses (SMI) most often include diagnoses of schizophrenia, bipolar disorder, and major depression. Recreational therapists working in adult behavioral health are likely to support individuals with these diagnoses. Consistent with the transdiagnostic approach, recreational therapists frequently work in groups serving a number of individuals with different diagnoses. Therefore, understanding how impairments in activities and participation may present differently across participants is important to the assessment process. For example, an impairment in handling stress and psychological demands (d240) may present as isolating behaviors in one individual, whereas it may present as aggressive behavior in someone else. In fact, Reed and colleagues (2009) suggest using the ICF checklists. The ICF checklist is a form that includes all domains and subdomains with checkboxes associated with scoring the entire ICF not as an independent assessment tool, but rather as a framework to document the consumer's functional status. By using direct observations and other standardized assessment tools, the ICF checklist may be a useful tool to synthesize the assessment process and provide guidance on setting observable, behavioral outcomes. In a study of 100 adults with anxiety, depression, and psychotic disorders, over 50 percent of participants in each diagnostic group reported severe impairments in the following areas in the Activities and Participation section of the ICF: problem solving; undertaking multiple tasks; conversation; housework; complex interpersonal relationships; relating to strangers; formal

TABLE 6.1 ICF Body Function Domains Relevant to RT Practice for Specific Diagnoses

Health condition	GLOBAL MENTAL FUNCTIONS		SPECIFIC MENTAL FUNCTIONS						DIGESTIVE, METABOLIC AND ENDOCRINE FUNCTIONS	GENITOURINARY & REPRODUCTIVE FUNCTIONS
	b126, Temperament and personality	b130, Energy and drive	**b140,** Attention	b144, Memory	b152, Emotion	**b160,** Thought	**b164,** Higher-level cognition	b180, Experience of self and time	b530, Weight maintenance	b640, Sexual Function
ADHD	X	X	X	X			X	X		
BD*	X	X	X	X	X	X	X		X	X
BPD	X	X			X			X		
MDD*	X	X	X	X	X	X	X	X	X	X
FED	X	X			X	X	X	X		
ODD	X		X		X					
PTSD	X	X	X	X	X	X		X		
SSD*	X	X	X	X	X	X	X	X	X	X
SUD	X	X			X					X

*ICF Core Set developed. ADHD: Attention deficit hyperactivity disorder; BD: bipolar disorder; BPD: borderline personality disorder; MDD: major depressive disorder; FED: feeding and eating disorders; ODD: oppositional defiant disorder and conduct disorder; PTSD: post-traumatic stress disorder; SSD: schizophrenia spectrum disorders; SUD: substance use disorders. **Codes in bold text represent identified transdiagnostic processes.**

TABLE 6.2 ICF Activities and Participation Domains Relevant to RT Practice for Specific Diagnoses

	D2, GENERAL TASKS AND DEMANDS		D5, SELF-CARE	D7, INTERPERSONAL INTERACTIONS			D8, MAJOR LIFE AREAS	D9, COMMUNITY, SOCIAL, AND CIVIC LIFE
	d230, Carrying out daily routine	d240, Handling stress	d570, Looking after one's health	d710, Basic interpersonal interactions	d720, Complex interpersonal interactions	d760, Family relationships	d845, Acquiring, keeping, terminating job	d920, Recreation and leisure
ADHD		X	X		X	X	X	X
BD*	X	X	X	X	X	X	X	X
BPD		X	X	X	X			
MDD*	X	X	X	X	X	X	X	X
FED		X	X	X	X	X		X
ODD		X			X			X
PTSD		X	X					X
SSD*	X	X	X	X	X	X	X	X
SUD	X	X	X	X	X	X	X	X

*ICF Core Set developed. ADHD: Attention deficit hyperactivity disorder; BD: bipolar disorder; BPD: borderline personality disorder; MDD: major depressive disorder; FED: feeding and eating disorders; ODD: oppositional defiant disorder and conduct disorder; PTSD: post-traumatic stress disorder; SSD: schizophrenia spectrum disorders; SUD: substance use disorders. **Codes in bold text represent identified transdiagnostic processes.**

TABLE 6.3   ICF Environment and Personal Domains Relevant to RT Practice for Specific Diagnoses

	E1, PRODUCTS AND TECHNOLOGY	E3, SUPPORT AND RELATIONSHIPS		E4, ATTITUDES			E5, SERVICES, SYSTEMS, AND POLICIES
	e1101, Drugs	e320, Friends	e355, Health professionals	e410, Attitudes of family members	e450, Attitudes of health professionals	e460, Societal attitudes	e580, Health services, systems, and policies
ADHD							
BD*	X	X	X	X	X	X	X
BPD					X		X
MDD*	X	X	X	X	X	X	X
FED	X	X	X	X		X	
ODD							
PTSD							
SSD*	X	X	X	X	X	X	X
SUD		X					

*ICF Core Set developed. ADHD: Attention deficit hyperactivity disorder; BD: bipolar disorder; BPD: borderline personality disorder; MDD: major depressive disorder; FED: feeding and eating disorders; ODD: oppositional defiant disorder and conduct disorder; PTSD: post-traumatic stress disorder; SSD: schizophrenia spectrum disorders; SUD: substance use disorders. **Codes in bold text represent identified transdiagnostic processes.**

relations; informal relations; family relationships; economic self-sufficiency; community life; and recreation/leisure (Tenorio-Martínez, del Carmen Lara-Muñoz, & Medina-Mora, 2009). The case study at the end of this chapter provides a narrative description of a case and treatment plan; following this, the related ICF codes and impairment are reported.

Standardized Assessment Tools

There are many assessment tools RTs use both in the development of individualized treatment plans and in communicating progress with the broader treatment team. These tools may be specific to RT or may be tools used across

disciplines. The following sections review tools that are external to RT and those developed specifically to use in RT practice. Familiarity with these tools and the process of reviewing additional tools in connection with the transdiagnostic approach will help RT professionals be more intentional about which assessment tools to use and how to communicate findings to other treatment team members and relevant stakeholders.

Tools External to RT

There are many assessment tools outside of recreational therapy that may be beneficial in the implementation of RT services. By increasing familiarity with these tools, recreational therapists have the opportunity to engage with broader disciplines and engage in an assessment process that includes outcome measures recommended by national mental health experts. The National Quality Forum (www.qualityforum.org/Qps/QpsTool.aspx), National Institutes of Health Toolbox (www.healthmeasures.net/explore-measurement-systems/nih-toolbox), and the PhenX toolkit (www.phenxtoolkit.org) are examples of resources that identify standardized assessment tools that have been evaluated and recommended by researchers. By selecting tools from these resources, recreational therapists can gain confidence that the identified tools meet the guidelines for best practices. Additionally, a number of these tools are free of charge and provide protocols for use. Following are descriptions of a number of assessment tools and how they relate to the transdiagnostic processes. This list is not exhaustive; however, the description of the tools will help the reader identify and evaluate additional tools.

Loneliness

The UCLA Loneliness measure is the most commonly used assessment to measure loneliness. The scale is included the PhenX toolkit, which is a National Institutes of Health (NIH)–funded project to identify broadly validated measures (Hamilton et al., 2011). This 20-item scale asks respondents to report on feelings about relationships, social support, and connectedness using a four-point scale ranging from *never* to *always*. Version 3 is the most current scale, with high reliability reported ranging from .89-.94 across three samples. The scale also has high convergent validity and construct validity (Russell, 1996). Creating and maintaining relationships are included across all three ICF core sets (i.e., schizophrenia spectrum disorders, major depressive disorder, bipolar disorder).

Loneliness may be an outcome of a variety of impairments in the processes identified. For example, loneliness may result from avoidance behaviors included under behavioral processes. Impairments in reasoning processes may make it difficult to interpret social stimuli, contributing to negative social experiences. Loneliness may also result from impairments in memory processing, particularly if individuals have difficulty recalling and making meaning from social experiences. Therefore, while loneliness is an important outcome for recreational therapists to measure, it is also important to assess the underlying processes that may contribute to the experience of loneliness.

Positive and Negative Emotions

The modified Differential Emotions Scale (mDES) is a 20-item measure used to assess one's experience of positive and negative emotions. Respondents are asked to identify the frequency of an emotion in the previous two weeks using a five-point scale ranging from *not at all* to *extremely often*. The score for the 10 positive emotions and the 10 negative emotions are totaled independently and divided by 10 to create an average positive and negative score (Fredrickson, Tugade, Waugh, & Larkin, 2003).

Positive and negative emotions are directly related to emotional processing. Understanding the level of negative and positive emotions experienced by clients can provide the insight necessary to develop interventions to decrease negative emotions and increase positive emotions. According to the Broaden and Build Theory of positive emotions, positive emotions serve as a resource that help individuals broaden their experiences and build problem-solving skills, whereas negative emotions force an individual to narrow his or her focus and limit creativity.

Disability Assessment

Developed by the World Health Organization, the World Health Organization Disability Assessment Schedule (WHODAS 2.0) is intended to measure health and disability across diagnostic groups and across cultures. This 36-item measure assesses six areas of functioning, including cognition, mobility, self-care, getting along, life activities, and participation. The WHODAS 2.0 has high test retest reliability, with intraclass correlations of the subscales ranging from .93-.96 and .98 for the entire measure. Among individuals with mental illnesses, subscale Cronbach's Alpha ranged from .92-94 and .98 for the entire measure, demonstrating high reliability when used in a behavioral health setting. The WHODAS 2.0 also has acceptable levels of concurrent validity and has demonstrated sensitivity to change when used as an outcome measure with individuals receiving treatment for depression (Üstün, Kostanjsek, Chatterji, & Rehm, 2010). This instrument is also found in the PhenX toolkit.

The WHODAS 2.0 measures a number of the processes identified in the transdiagnostic approach as well as areas identified by the NIH. The cognition subscale targets the participant's perspective of difficulty with communication and thinking activities, including concentration, memory, problem solving, learning, and communicating. The mobility section is related to the motor tasks identified by the NIH. The getting along subscale targeting relationships assesses difficulty an individual has had in both close relationships and interacting with strangers. This domain not only connects to social relationships, which is identified in the emotions domain of the NIH toolkit, but it also connects to the behavioral processes within the transdiagnostic approach. The remaining subscales (self-care, getting along, life activities, and participation) relate to sensation (identified by NIH) and the behavioral processes presented in the transdiagnostic approach.

Tools Internal to RT

In terms of areas of practice, behavioral and mental health is the single largest area of employment for recreational therapists, representing the practice setting for 37 percent of all recreational therapists with the CTRS credential (National Council for Therapeutic Recreation Certification, 2014). As such, it is somewhat surprising how few standardized RT assessments have been created for the behavioral and mental health area of practice. Of the 17 standardized functional skill assessment instruments listed in Burlingame and Blaschko's (2010) *Assessment in Therapeutic Recreation* (4th edition), only three instruments are specifically noted as applicable to the behavioral and mental health setting.

One of the first developed assessment instruments specifically designed for use in behavioral and mental health services is the Comprehensive Evaluation in Recreational Therapy—Psych/Behavioral, Revised (CERT-Psych/R; Burlingame & Blaschko,

2010). Among recreational therapists practicing in mental health settings, just over 9 percent report using the CERT-Psych/R (Kemeny et al., 2016). Initially created by Parker and colleagues in 1975 (as cited in Burlingame & Blaschko, 2010), this instrument is used to record data on a client's behavior in general, as well as in individual and group performance. General functional behaviors include such things as attendance and appearance, as well as attitude toward RT services. Individual performance focuses on cognitive and emotional functional skills such as attention span, decision making, judgment, expression of hostility, and frustration tolerance, as well as performance in activities principally reflecting abilities to organize and initiate behavior. Group performance focuses on behaviors related to interpersonal function such as leadership ability, group conversation, handling of interpersonal conflict, interpersonal competitiveness, interpersonal interaction, and conversation. Although the CERT has been available and utilized in RT services for more than 40 years, there is very little information available on either its reliability or validity (Burlingame & Blaschko, 2010).

Another assessment instrument identified as appropriate for behavioral and psychiatric practice is the Therapeutic Recreation Activity Assessment (TRAA; Burlingame & Blaschko, 2010). This instrument is used to collect data on functional skills as demonstrated in a group setting. The TRAA appears to be the most commonly used standardized instrument, with almost 14 percent of RTs in mental health practice reporting using it for assessment (Kemeny et al., 2016). The TRAA collects data on fine motor skills, gross motor skills, receptive communication, expressive communication, cognitive skills, and social behaviors. The assessment is completed through observation of clients while undertaking three tasks involving 1) a card matching game, 2) simple nonstrenuous physical exercises, and 3) an arts and crafts project. The TRAA has been evaluated for content validity based on expert review and interrater reliability is reported at 92 percent (Burlingame & Blaschko, 2010).

The Functional Assessment for Characteristics for Therapeutic Recreation, Revised (FAC-

TR-R) was first developed in 1983 by Peterson, Dunn, and Carruthers (as cited in Burlingame & Blaschko, 2010) to provide a basis for recreational specialists without formal training as a therapist to identify areas of functional need that could be addressed through recreational therapy (Burlingame & Blaschko, 2010). The FACTR-R is used to collect data on 11 aspects of functioning in the physical, cognitive, and social/emotional domains. Burlingame and Blaschko noted that the FACTR-R is not a testing tool, but instead characterized it as a screening tool that is useful in identifying areas to address through recreational therapy. The FACTR-R has no reported validity or reliability analyses.

CASE STUDY

ICF Coding for Behavioral Health

The following case presents Art, a man who was receiving mental health services through a community mental health center Assertive Community Treatment (ACT) team. As you are reading through the case, use the following ICF coding sheet to identify areas of assessment relevant to the ICF as well as the transdiagnostic processes.

ICF CODING SHEET

BODY FUNCTIONS

Code/impairment	Description
Mental functions	
Voice and speech functions	

ACTIVITIES AND PARTICIPATION

Code/impairment	Description
Learning and applying knowledge	
General tasks/demands	

> continued

CASE STUDY   *> continued*

ACTIVITIES AND PARTICIPATION (*continued*)

Code/impairment	Description
Communications	
Mobility	
Interpersonal relationships	
Community life	

ENVIRONMENTAL FACTORS

Code/impairment	Description
Products and technology	
Support and relationships	
Services, systems, and policies	

Overview and Assessment

Art is a 51-year-old male diagnosed with schizophrenia. He is from rural Missouri and has lived in his community for the past 10 years, moving there because of the availability of mental health services. Art requires medication delivery twice a day, at which time the case worker will also ensure he drinks a high calorie nutritional shake. Beyond the nutritional shake, Art's diet consists mostly of sweets. Art has two sisters in the state who visit about once a month. His only other interaction is with mental health providers. Art has a roommate with whom he has little interaction. He also experiences negative symptoms (e.g., alogia, amotivation, anhedonia, asociality, blunted affect) and cognitive dysfunction, resulting in severe impairments in communication, including both written and verbal communication. Art also has severe impairments in planning and initiating behavior, spending most of his days in bed.

Art lives in semi-independent living housing owned by the mental health agency, where he and a roommate reside. He does not demonstrate the ability to independently shop for or prepare simple meals. Additionally, he requires prompting and assistance to maintain clean and orderly personal and shared space within his home. Art needs assistance with instrumental activities of daily living, including personal hygiene, cooking, cleaning, shopping for and preparing meals, and eating a balanced diet. His difficulty with independently scheduling his day makes it challenging for him to complete ADLs or to participate in enjoyable activities.

At assessment, Art had limited perceived competence to access his community independently. He is scared of getting lost and unwilling to go places he is not 100 percent sure he can find. This means that he is only comfortable walking to the grocery store (1.5 blocks down the street) and Bridges Mental Health Center (next door). Art has no set weekly schedule and seems to spend almost all day in bed. He does not identify any activities or places that he goes to or enjoys going to in his town other than the grocery store and Bridges. He says he has used the bus before, but does not enjoy it and is often confused about which bus to take. Art can go to the grocery store independently, but does not independently access the community for other goods and services.

Art has limited daily social interactions as well as limited opportunity for social interactions. Social interactions he does have consist of limited conversations with his roommate and conversations with mental health professionals. He did not express a desire for more friendships; however, he enjoys when people stop by. Art says that he is friends with his roommate, but they do not talk very much, if at all. He did not mention desiring a romantic relationship. Art misses his siblings and enjoys when he gets to see them. He wants to go back home to the country because that is where his family is. Art is not assertive with strangers. He has a history of giving money to strangers that come by his residence.

Art is of average weight, but does not have healthy eating patterns. He requires prompting to eat food beyond sweets. His physician has told him he needs to exercise daily, and he is working to do so. He enjoys walking, but is afraid of getting lost.

Using a picture assessment developed for a research study to assess interest in recreational activities, as well as perceived barriers and facilitators of participation, Art identified interest in walking, sewing, watching TV, and playing board games with friends. Art showed the recreational therapist a broken sewing machine and pants quilt he had begun making.

Recreational Therapy Interventions

Using a strengths-based approach, in which Art's interests and skills are the basis for planning, Art and the recreational therapist codeveloped the following treatment plan.

The recreational therapist will meet with Art three times a week for a minimum of 45 minutes each time. During these times, the recreational therapist will work with Art on the following areas:

1. **Scheduling and daily activity engagement:** The recreational therapist will work with Art to incorporate a picture schedule into his daily routine. Together, they will identify daily goals and activities, creating pictures that represent the activities. Activities will include (but are not limited to) medication, eating, and personal hygiene. The daily picture schedule will be on a Velcro calendar, and once completed, Art will move each activity to a completed column to reinforce independent engagement. The picture schedule will be introduced to the rest of the Assertive Community Treatment (ACT) team so the team members delivering medication

> continued

in the mornings and evenings are able to prompt him about his activity engagement. This component of the intervention will support Art to improve his higher-level cognition (b164) and carry out his daily routine (d230).

2. **Communication:** Art will talk with the recreational therapist about his day. He will respond to questions about his emotional experience. The recreational therapist will use open-ended questions to encourage conversation. Art will work toward initiating conversation. Therapists on his treatment team will reinforce Art's social skills in both initiating and maintaining conversation. This includes interactions with the therapist as well as members of his social network and other social interactions. These activities will support Art to improve his basic and complex interpersonal interactions (d710; d720).

3. **Walking:** Art will walk with the recreational therapist twice a week on the nearby trail. At the end of 10 weeks, Art will walk 1.5 miles independently twice a week. During these walks, the recreational therapist will work with Art to identify meaningful landmarks to support independent navigation and reduce his fear of getting lost. These activities support Art's weight maintenance (b530) and his ability to look after his own health (d570). Encouraging independent participation promotes motivation (b130) and community participation (d920).

4. **Sewing:** Art will independently work on his blanket daily. He will demonstrate progress to the recreational therapist after walks. The recreational therapist will work with Art to learn how to problem solve issues with his sewing machine. Like walking, his work on sewing increases motivation and participation in leisure activities (b130; d920).

Summary

Assessment is an important part of the RT process. Beyond collecting information about clients, the assessment process allows RTs to interpret information about an individual's strengths, barriers, facilitators, and functioning. Understanding the transdiagnostic approach to assessment gives RTs working in behavioral health a common understanding of areas of functioning that may be affected across diagnostic groups. Similarly, the common language used in both the transdiagnostic approach and the ICF allows the RT practitioner to be an equal player with other disciplines when communicating with the entire treatment team. When conducting assessments, RT practitioners should consider both standardized assessments within RT and those that are common across behavioral health service delivery. When considering new assessments, RT practitioners should evaluate tools based on their applicability within the desired setting and its relationship to the areas of functioning common across diagnostic groupings.

REFLECTION QUESTIONS

1. How does the ICF improve upon the use of historical domains of assessment such as cognitive, physical, social, emotional, and leisure?

2. What is the basic concept underlying a transdiagnostic approach to RT behavioral health practice?

3. Of the transdiagnostic processes identified within the ICF's domain of specific mental functions, which one has been identified in almost all diagnoses examined in this chapter?

4. Of the transdiagnostic processes identified within the ICF's domain of activities and participation, which one has been identified within all diagnoses examined in this chapter?

5. Which behavioral health diagnoses have established ICF Core Sets?

6. What are two sources of publicly available assessment instruments that can be used in recreational therapy behavioral health practice?

7. Of the standardized assessment tools internal to recreational therapy, which one is the most commonly used by practitioners in behavioral health?

8. Based on the case study, what is one area of mental function in which Art demonstrates a limitation?

9. Based on the case study, what is one area of activities and participation in which Art demonstrates a limitation?

REFERENCES

Austin, D.R., & McCormick, B.P. (2013). Clinical reasoning: A concept for recreational therapy. *American Journal of Recreational Therapy, 12*(4).

Barlow, D.H. (2011). *Unified protocol for transdiagnostic treatment of emotional disorders: Therapist guide.* New York: Oxford University Press.

Becker, E.S., Margraf, J., Türke, V., Soeder, U., & Neumer, S. (2001). Obesity and mental illness in a representative sample of young women. *International Journal of Obesity and Related Metabolic Disorders, 25 Suppl 1*, S5-9. doi:10.1038/sj.ijo.0801688

Brown, T.A., & Barlow, D.H. (2009). A proposal for a dimensional classification system based on the shared features of the DSM-IV anxiety and mood disorders: Implications for assessment and treatment. *Psychological Assessment, 21*(3), 256-271. doi:10.1037/a0016608

Burlingame, J., & Blaschko, T.M. (2010). *Assessment tools for recreational therapy and related fields.* Enumclaw, WA: Idyll Arbor.

Fredrickson, B.L., Tugade, M.M., Waugh, C.E., & Larkin, G.R. (2003). What good are positive emotions in crises? A prospective study of resilience and emotions following the terrorist attacks on the United States on September 11th, 2001. *Journal of Personality and Social Psychology, 84*(2), 365-376.

Hamilton, C.M., Strader, L.C., Pratt, J.G., Maiese, D., Henderohot, T., Kwok, R.K., et al. (2011). The PhenX toolkit: Get the most from your measures. *American Journal of Epidemiology, 174*(3), 253-260. doi:10.1093/aje/kwr193

Harvey, A.G., Watkins, E., Mansell, W., & Shafran, R. (2004). *Cognitive behavioural processes across psychological disorders: A transdiagnostic approach to research and treatment.* New York: Oxford University Press.

Hasson-Ohayon, I., Arnon-Ribenfeld, N., Hamm, J., & Lysaker, P. (2017, September). Agency before action: The application of behavioral activation in psychotherapy with persons with psychosis. *Psychotherapy, 54*(3), 245-254. http://dx.doi.org/10.1037/pst0000114

Hunsley, J., & Mash, E.J. (2007). Evidence-based assessment. *Annual Review of Clinical Psychology, 3*, 29-51. doi:10.1146/annurev.clinpsy.3.022806.091419

Kemeny, M.E., Hutchins, D., & Cooke, C.A. (2016). Current status of assessment in recreational therapy practice. *American Journal of Recreational Therapy, 15*(4), 11-21. doi:10.5055/ajrt.2016.0115

Kessler, R.C., Chiu, W.T., Demler, O., Merikangas, K.R., & Walters, E.E. (2005). Prevalence, severity, and comorbidity of 12-month DSM-IV disorders in the national comorbidity survey replication. *Archives of General Psychiatry, 62*(6), 617-627. doi:10.1001/archpsyc.62.6.617

Kring, A.M., & Sloan, D.M. (2010). *Emotion regulation and psychopathology: A transdiagnostic approach to etiology and treatment.* New York: Guilford Press.

Millan, M.J., Agid, Y., Bruene, M., Bullmore, E.T., Carter, C.S., Clayton, N.S., et al. (2012). Cognitive dysfunction in psychiatric disorders: Characteristics, causes and the quest for improved therapy. *Nature Reviews Drug Discovery, 11*, 141-168. doi:10.1038/nrd3628

National Council for Therapeutic Recreation Certification. (2014). CTRS® professional profile. Retrieved from https://nctrc.org/wp-content/uploads/2015/02/MM2-ctrs-professional-profile-brochure.pdf

Neely, K., Parker, D., & Campbell, J. (2015). Post-traumatic stress disorder. In H.R. Porter (Ed.), *Recreational therapy for specific diagnoses and conditions* (pp. 309-320). Enumclaw, WA: Idyll Arbor.

Porter, H.R. (2015a). Attention-deficit/hyperactivity disorder. In H.R. Porter (Ed.), *Recreational therapy for specific diagnoses and conditions* (pp. 27-37). Enumclaw, WA: Idyll Arbor.

Porter, H.R. (Ed.). (2015b). *Recreational therapy for specific diagnoses and conditions.* Enumclaw, WA: Idyll Arbor.

Reed, G.M., Leonardi, M., Ayuso-Mateos, J.L., Materzanini, A., Castronuovo, D., Manara, A., et al. (2009). Implementing the ICF in a psychiatric rehabilitation setting for people with serious mental illness in the Lombardy region of Italy. *Disability and Rehabilitation, 31 Suppl 1,* S170-173.

Russell, D.W. (1996). UCLA loneliness scale (version 3): Reliability, validity, and factor structure. *Journal of Personality Assessment, 66*(1), 20-40. doi:10.1207/s15327752jpa6601_2

Schwalberg, M.D., Barlow, D.H., Alger, S.A., & Howard, L.J. (1992). Comparison of bulimics, obese binge eaters, social phobics, and individuals with panic disorder on comorbidity across DSM-III-R anxiety disorders. *Journal of Abnormal Psychology, 101*(4), 675-681.

Seligman, M.E.P. (1991). *Learned optimism.* New York: A.A. Knopf.

Tenorio-Martínez, R., del Carmen Lara-Muñoz, M., & Medina-Mora, M.E. (2009). Measurement of problems in activities and participation in patients with anxiety, depression and schizophrenia using the ICF checklist. *Social Psychiatry and Psychiatric Epidemiology, 44*(5), 377-384. doi:10.1007/s00127-008-0449-3

Üstün, T.B., Kostanjsek, N., Chatterji, S., & Rehm, J. (2010). *Measuring health and disability: Manual for WHO disability assessment schedule WHODAS 2.0.* Geneva: World Health Organization.

Werner, K., & Gross, J.J. (2010). Emotion regulation and psychopathology: A conceptual framework. In A.M. Kring & D.M. Sloan (Eds.), *Emotion regulation and psychopathology: A transdiagnostic approach to etiology and treatment* (pp. 13-37). New York: Guilford Press.

Wood, S., Wyble, J.R., & Charters, J. (2015). Substance use disorders. In H.R. Porter (Ed.), *Recreational therapy for specific diagnoses* (pp. 385-398). Enumclaw, WA: Idyll Arbor.

World Health Organization. (2001). ICF: *International classification of functioning, disability and health.* Geneva: Author.

Yang, H., & Payne, M.P. (2015). Oppositional defiant disorder and conduct disorder. In H.R. Porter (Ed.), *Recreational therapy for specific diagnoses* (pp. 269-276). Enumclaw, WA: Idyll Arbor.

Zemishlany, Z., & Weizman, A. (2008). The impact of mental illness on sexual dysfunction. *Advances in Psychosomatic Medicine, 29,* 89-106. doi:10.1159/000126626

ADDITIONAL RESOURCES

Austin, D.R. (2013). *Therapeutic recreation processes & techniques: Evidence-based recreational therapy.* Champaign, IL: Sagamore.

CHAPTER 7

Assessment of Outcomes in Physical Disability: Considerations and Recommendations for Recreational Therapy

David P. Loy, PhD, LRT/CTRS

LEARNING OBJECTIVES

Upon completion of the text, the student will demonstrate:

- Knowledge of evidence-based recreational therapy assessment instruments used to determine functioning of individuals with physical disabilities.

- Knowledge of the impact of limitations in physical, cognitive, social, and emotional functioning on the ability to determine the functioning of individuals with physically disabling conditions.

- Knowledge of evidence-based assessment instruments from other health care disciplines that may be relevant to recreational therapy practice when assessing physical functioning.

- Knowledge of the World Health Organization's (WHO) *International Classification of Functioning, Disability and Health* (ICF) as a method of classifying individual functioning and the impact of activity limitations and restrictions to participation in life activities, independence, satisfaction, and quality of life.

The World Health Organization (WHO, 2017) indicates that approximately 15 percent of the world's population has some form of disability. Included in these numbers are many individuals with physical disabilities that limit their ability to function independently within their communities. The recreational therapist needs to develop assessment competencies that provide information for the treatment of these individuals. The ICF classifies many of the health and health-related domains relevant to the treatment of individuals with physical disabilities (WHO, 2017). This chapter provides the reader information about the assessment of individuals with physically disabling conditions, as well as information about the identification, implementation, and interpretation of specific assessment instruments that recreational therapists use to directly measure ICF functional outcomes for individuals with physical disabilities.

Purpose of Assessment in Physical Disability

A recreational therapist utilizes a wide range of activity and community based interventions and techniques to enhance the "physical, cognitive, emotional, social, and leisure development of their clients" (ATRA, 2019). However, the ability to improve the needs of clients revolves around the ability to assess and identify those outcomes that require interventions (Stumbo, 2003). While the recreational therapist serves a variety of populations, individuals with physical disabilities may provide the most varied needs requiring effective assessment.

Safety and Readiness for Treatment

Often, participants in recreational therapy may not be ready for program involvement. The use of sound, valid assessment techniques can provide the therapist the information needed to determine if treatment is appropriate for a participant with a physical disability. Does the patient have the ability to sit up long enough for active treatment? What is the patient's current level of pain, and will he or she be able to tolerate a recreational therapy session? Therapists often employ simple screening assessments to determine if an individual is medically ready to participate in treatment sessions.

Establishing a Baseline

There is certainly more emphasis than in the past on the use of evidence-based interventions in allied health (Skalko, Sauter, Burgess, & Loy, 2013). The effectiveness of interventions is determined by the ability of the researcher or practitioner to demonstrate a therapeutic change in a participant's outcome. Sound assessment and measurement techniques provide a baseline to compare the impact of a particular recreational therapy intervention. Therapeutic change is impossible to determine without comparative measurement points established by the recreational therapist.

Program Placement

The ultimate goal of recreational therapy assessment is to provide data necessary to place individuals in the most appropriate program (Stumbo & Peterson, 2009). Valid and effective assessment of individuals with physical disabilities assists the recreational therapist in placing individuals in the appropriate treatment program based on the determined level of function. The recreational therapist can also use information obtained in an assessment to compare to established normative data to determine if the client is below the norm, at the norm, or above the norm. This information can assist the therapist in determining the need and subsequent placement of the client in a program. For example, the recreational therapist may administer the Timed Up and Go (TUG) test and determine that the individual performs at a higher time score but within the normative time range for someone his or her age. The recreational therapist then has confidence to place the client in a standing exercise group rather than a seated exercise group.

Program Evaluation and Research

Evaluating programs is essential in determining the composition of programs within an agency's comprehensive program. Recreational therapy managers must provide continuous program evaluation to determine efficiencies and effectiveness. Valid assessment of interventions can help determine which specific programs are effective in promoting the targeted and intended therapeutic outcome (Stumbo & Peterson, 2009). Intervention programs for individuals with physical disabilities that fail to collect and measure outcome data resulting from such interventions have limited knowledge to continue offering such programs. Similarly, researchers investigating recreational therapy interventions need to use valid assessment protocols to determine the ability of an intervention to change targeted outcomes in a therapeutic direction (ATRA, 2019). Research, in its purest form, can and does provide valuable information for recreational therapists to evaluate the efficacy of programs (Stumbo & Peterson, 2009).

Physical Assessment Competencies for Recreational Therapists

The recreational therapist must have certain competencies that permit the effective assessment of individuals with physical disabilities. These competencies result from opportunities to learn and practice those skills essential to the assessment of individuals with physical disabilities. There are many reasons why recreational therapists must establish such assessment competencies.

Conceptualization and Operationalization

The recreational therapist must have an accurate idea of what he or she is measuring to ensure the physical outcome is valid for the client being served. The word *construct* is often used to depict concepts that are abstract or broadly defined such as aggression, love, or even pain. The *conceptualization* of a construct provides a better understanding of the outcome, or construct, through a historical series of theoretical research established from a series of related literature. While consistencies within the literature help formulate a coherent conceptualization of the outcome or construct being measured, there are often new investigations that challenge the current conceptualization of an outcome.

While it is important to understand the concepts being measured, it is even more critical for the recreational therapist to be able to operationalize the concept being measured. *Operationalization* is the way a practitioner or researcher links a concept to more concrete and tangible indicators that can be collected through statistical measurements (Stumbo, 2003). For example, the concept of pain is a theoretical concept that we often operationalize in numerical ways by asking a client to assess their pain on a scale of 1 to 10. Therefore, pain in this example is operationalized as anything greater than zero and the perceived levels can be captured in degrees or statistical units to help the practitioner better operationalize the degree to which the client is experiencing pain. Operationalization of outcomes provides a better way of measuring and ultimately understanding the concept.

Measurement

Measurement is the process of systematically assigning numbers to objects and their properties in order to accurately depict and describe an object (Burlingame & Blaschko, 2010). For example, one could easily portray the role of the local fair vendor and guess someone's weight, but the assigning of numbers to how much one weighs is only accomplished through the accurate measurement through a set of rules we use to measure outcomes. Measurement of RT outcomes in clients with physical disabilities often includes performance tests, observation scoring, or even client survey administration. The recreational therapist must possess the ability to produce consistent results through application of these measurement protocols that provide a system of collecting data. Inconsistencies within such measurement protocols challenge the validity and reliability of such results. Therefore, it is critical for the recreational therapist to develop measurement competencies that produce consistent and accurate results with those physical properties being assessed.

Interpretation

Once the therapist has accurately measured the outcome, they must then provide an interpretation of the status of the particular client. *Interpretation* of the assessment includes the ability of the recreational therapist to translate statistical outcome data to determine if the client is below, at, or above established standards. An accurate interpretation of the collected physical outcome data will have an impact on the specific treatment plan (Stumbo & Peterson, 2009). Certainly, the recreational therapist can use his or her clinical judgment, expertise, or clinical reasoning to interpret the outcomes collected (Burlingame & Blaschko, 2010). Comparing results of physical outcome data collection to normative data samples can provide the therapist a more informed way to interpret the status of his or her client. For example, a therapist determines that her client, a 70-year-old female, has hand grip strength measured at 18 pounds in her right hand. When the therapist compares this data to normative standards (Mathiowetz, Weber, Volland, & Kashman, 1984), she determines that her patient's right hand grip strength is below the normative standards of 33 to 78 pounds for a 70-year-old woman. She can then develop a treatment plan that focuses on appropriate strength training. Comparing results of phys-

ical outcome measurement data to normative standards provides the recreational therapist information to accurately interpret assessment of the client.

Use of Documentation and Health Care Records

Finally, the ability to write and use existing documentation is another important competency necessary for the recreational therapist to accurately measure clients with physically disabling conditions. Some feel the assessment process begins at the initial moment you come in contact with the client. However, it is important for the therapist to collect valuable data prior to the initial meeting with the client. For example, the therapist should develop a habit of collecting premeeting information through a review of the client's health care records. Specific data collected by other allied health team members such as physical, occupational, and speech therapists can provide the recreational therapist important data that will expedite the assessment process and often put a meaningful context to data collected during the RT assessment. Sharing of interdisciplinary team data is important to providing a holistic assessment of the client with physical disabilities. Beyond the preassessment data, the recreational therapist needs to develop competencies to document results, interpretations, and recommendations within the medical chart to establish a historical record of the client's outcome assessment.

Assessment and Measurement Issues in Physical Disability

Valid assessment and measurement of physical outcomes in individuals with physical disabilities can provide a foundation for the establishment of appropriate treatment goals that provide effective treatment options. However, the very attributes being measured can also create difficulties in assessment and may even challenge the accuracy of the data collected by the recreational therapist. It is important for the recreational therapist to understand some of those attributes that can make the assessment process more difficult.

Physical Limitations

Some assessment protocols may require the client to physically perform a test. However, many disability groups served by recreational therapists have physical limitations that affect the ability to perform various assessment tests. Clients can have visual or hearing impairments that limit administration of particular instruments. To accommodate, the therapist may need to read aloud instructions, increase font size of words and symbols, provide instructions in a written format, or use contrasting colors to better allow reading of assessment materials. If the client is unable to stand due to limited strength or gross motor function in their lower extremities, the performance test to measure balance may not be appropriate for the client, or adaptations may need to be made. This test includes both standing and sitting protocols, and normative standards for both sitting and standing administration are provided for therapist interpretation.

Cognitive Limitations

Assessment often requires the client to understand the measurement protocols and/or answer particular questions in the assessment. Many clients served by recreational therapists have cognitive limitations that may limit the ability to understand or perform such tests. It is important for the therapist to explain the instructions clearly and break down the tasks in the most basic way to promote cognitive understanding. The test may not even be cognitively appropriate, based on typical developmental milestones. For example, a child may not have the cognitive ability to assess their pain with a numerical scale. Therefore, pediatric pain scales using images of facial expressions have been used to better assess pain in children (Wong-Baker FACES Foundation, 2016). If the therapist questions the validity of the results based on the cognitive status of the client, it may be necessary to use techniques to further validate such performance tests. The therapist can confirm, or triangulate, their results by comparing collected results with other rehabilitation team members, discussing results with family members familiar with the functional abilities of the client, or checking historical trends captured over the duration of treatment to identify potential outliers and the realistic consistency of results.

Communication Limitations

Finally, the client may lack certain skills needed to perform assessments due to an inability to communicate. For those with deficits in communication skills due to cerebrovascular accidents (CVA) or cerebral palsy (CP), the therapist may need to incorporate communication boards, pointers, or communication cards in the assessment process. In addition, the recreational therapist should also understand cultural differences that may influence the assessment of outcomes in clients with physical disabilities. For example, individuals from different cultural backgrounds may not comprehend instructions or the cultural and contextual use of some words used in the assessment process. The therapist should consider using interpreters or image-based instructions or adopting use of assessments with valid versions in the preferred language of the client.

Altering the Assessment Protocol for Individuals With Physical Disabilities

Sometimes it may be necessary to adapt assessment protocols based on the physical needs of clients with disabilities. However, it should be pointed out that when validated protocols are changed, the psychometric evidence is no longer supportive since the procedures were not the same as those validated. The recreational therapist often has to make a judgment about whether altering published assessment protocols is necessary to allow the client with physical disabilities to perform the test and therefore produce the most valid results possible. Even when altered protocols are used, the RT professional can continue to use them to track a client's treatment progress, as long as the same exact protocol is used in a pre-post test method (NCHPAD, 2017).

Connection to *International Classification of Functioning, Disability and Health*

The concepts and terminology used by the *International Classification of Functioning, Disability and Health* (ICF) are important to the practice, education, research, and training of recreational therapists (ATRA, 2019). In October of 2005, the American Therapeutic Recreation Association (ATRA) adopted the use of the ICF classification and coding system in RT practice, including the assessment of clients. This chapter will utilize the ICF classification structure to provide outcomes and instruments used in the assessment of individuals with physical disabilities.

Measurement of Body Function

The ICF conceptualization of body functions includes the physiological function of the body systems. Many body functions are affected directly or indirectly by the impact of physical disability (Stumbo & Peterson, 2009). This section will list some of those body function classifications, including sensory functions, cardiovascular systems, and neuromusculoskeletal and movement-related functions and the respective assessment instruments that measure them.

Sensory Functions

About 15 million people have difficulty with sensory issues including seeing and hearing, including 2.0 million who are legally blind and 1.1 million individuals with severe hearing loss (U.S. Census Bureau, 2010). There are many physical disability groups served by recreational therapists that have sensory issues, including individuals with visual limitations, patients experiencing cerebrovascular accidents (CVA), aging individuals, clients with developmental disabilities, and individuals with hearing limitations. Recreational therapists are not the primary assessor of sensory outcomes in some settings, but it remains necessary for the recreational therapist to have knowledge of sensory issues as they relate to program involvement.

Seeing Functions (b210)

Seeing function is "sensory functions relating to sensing the presence of light and sensing the form, size, shape and color of the visual stimuli" (WHO, 2001, p. 62). Seeing function is assessed by a licensed vision health care provider, but it is certainly important for the recreational therapist to be able to interpret vision function for programmatic purposes. Individuals with physically disabling conditions have many vision functions classified in the ICF, including visual acuity, distance vision, ocular preference, and visual field function.

Visual Acuity Functions (b2100) Visual acuity is "seeing functions of sensing form and contour, both binocular and monocular, for both distant and near vision" (WHO, 2001, p. 62). Although the recreational therapist is not the primary assessor of visual acuity, it is important to understand the vision assessment process for interpretation and RT program placement and adaptation. One's vision classification is important to individuals with physical disabilities, because any person with vision that cannot be corrected to better than 20/200 in the best eye or who has 20 degrees (diameter) or less of visual field remaining is

TABLE 7.1 Classification of Vision Function

Degree of vision loss	Visual acuity
Normal vision	20/20-20/30
Moderate visual impairment	20/70-20/160
Severe visual impairment	20/200-20/1000
Blindness	more than 20/1000

Based on L. Dandona and R. Dandona, "Revision of Visual Impairment Definitions in the International Statistical Classification of Diseases," *BMC Medicine* 4 (2006): 7. https://www.ncbi.nlm.nih.gov/pmc/articles/PMC1435919/

considered legally blind or eligible for disability classification and possible inclusion in certain government-sponsored programs (see table 7.1).

Binocular (b21000) or Monocular (b21001) Activity of Distant Vision

Farsightedness is "seeing functions of sensing size, form and contour, using right/left or both eyes, for objects distant from the eye" (WHO, 2001, p. 62). While a licensed vision care provider administers a vision assessment through the use of the Snellen Eye Chart, the recreational therapist should be aware of how to interpret distance vision when expressed in a fraction where "20/20" is the standard of good/normal vision. In this fraction, the top number represents the distance one can see at the distance listed on bottom of someone with "normal" vision (WHO, 2017). Therefore, 20/100 means someone can see clear images at 20 feet where someone with good vision can see the same image at 100 feet. The use of the Snellen Eye Chart requires the individual to know the alphabet, thus limiting it to preschool pediatric populations. Therefore, eye charts for illiterate populations were developed, such as the Graham Field Kindergarten Eye Chart (www.grahamfield.com). Another vision function important for RT programming includes eye dominance.

Ocular Preference

Ocular preference, or eye dominance, is the tendency to prefer visual input from one eye as opposed to the other (Eser, Durrie, Schwendeman, & Stahl, 2008). Approximately two-thirds of the population is right-eye dominant and one-third left-eye dominant (Eser et al., 2008). A person is said to have *unilateral ocular preference* when the individual's dominant eye is on the same side as their dominant hand. Conversely, an individual is said to have *cross-dominance ocular preference* when the individual's dominant eye is on the opposite side as their dominant hand. Mann, Runswick, and Allen (2016) suggested that cricket players with cross-dominance ocular preference had an advantage because of the side-on stances. While there are multiple ways to assess eye dominance, the easiest way is the Miles Eye Dominance Test (Miles, 1930): The individual extends both arms, brings both hands together and connects index fingers and thumbs to create a triangle. With both eyes open, the individual views a distant object through the opening and then alternates closing the eyes. The dominant eye is the eye for which the object stays within the triangle when the other is closed.

Visual Field Functions (b2101)

Visual field function is defined as "seeing functions related to the entire area that can be seen with fixation of gaze" (WHO, 2001, p. 63). Visual field function is particularly important for individuals with physical disabilities who have had damage to one side of the brain, including stroke or brain injury. When one side of the brain is damaged, a condition called *unilateral neglect* (UN) can occur, wherein the individual is unaware of half of their visual field. The most common type of unilateral neglect is left spatial neglect, when an individual has damage to the right hemisphere of the brain and there is a lack of awareness of one's left visual field.

Right spatial neglect is rare because there is redundant processing of the right space by both the left and right cerebral hemispheres, whereas in most left-dominant brains the left space is only processed by the right cerebral hemisphere (Chen, Hreha, Fotis, Goedert, & Barrett, 2012).

Although there are more than 60 tests of spatial neglect, only half of those have been validated (Azouvi, Bartolomea, Beis, Perennou, Pradat-Diehl, & Rousseaux, 2006). Many of the assessments for UN require drawing, which highlights an absence or distortion of the left side of objects. Copying simple figures and free drawing are frequently used by therapists to detect UN in patients following stroke. Figures typically used for copying include flowers, stars, cubes, and geometric shapes. Test objects considered to be sensitive to detecting UN are a clock face, the human form, and a butterfly. Incomplete drawing or copying with omissions or gross distortions on the affected visual side is considered indicative of UN. In some situations, the person may confine the drawing to the unaffected side of the page (Plummer, Morris, & Dunai, 2003). One such drawing test is the Comprehensive Visual Neglect Assessment (CVNA), which was formerly known as Bond Howard Assessment on Neglect in Recreational Therapy (BARNT) (Burlingame & Blaschko, 2010). The CVNA measures the density and scope of visual neglect by incorporating drawing tasks in a dartboard chart.

Azouvi and colleagues (2006) suggested most tests for UN include a battery of quantitative tests, including paper-and-pencil tests, an assessment of personal neglect, and a behavioral assessment using the Catherine Bergego Scale (CBS) (Bergego, Azouvi, Samuel, Marchal, Louis-Dreyfus, Jokic, et al., 1995). The CBS is an observation assessment on a four-point scale (e.g., 0 = no neglect, 3 = severe neglect) of patient performance in 10 different real-life situations, including grooming, dressing, or wheelchair driving. High scores on the CBS (range = 0-30) reflect more difficulty with spatial neglect.

Hearing Functions (b230)

The ICF defines hearing function as "sensory functions relating to sensing the presence of sounds and discriminating the location, pitch, loudness and quality of sounds" (WHO, 2001, p. 65). About 7.6 million people report difficulty hearing, with approximately 1.1 million of those classified as having severe hearing loss (U.S. Census Bureau, 2010). While there are many specific aspects of hearing, the most appropriate for the RT might be the loudness of sound detected (as measured in decibels [dB]). During a hearing test performed by a trained audiologist, the assessment of sound detection is measured in the loudness of the sound (dB) when an individual *first* detects it. When an individual can only detect *higher* levels of sound loudness, there is a higher measure of hearing loss. Hearing loss is indicated within seven range levels (table 7.2).

TABLE 7.2   Degree of Hearing Loss Levels

Degree of hearing loss	Sound loudness at *initial* detection (dB)
Normal	−10 to 15
Slight	16 to 25
Mild	26 to 40
Moderate	41 to 55
Moderately severe	56 to 70
Severe	71 to 90
Profound	91+

Reprinted by permission from J.C. Clark, "Uses and abuses of hearing loss classification," *ASHA* 23 (1981): 492, table 2.

It is certainly outside the scope of practice for recreational therapists to assess and determine the sensitivity of hearing loss in clients. Those clinical assessments should be determined by licensed speech and language pathologists and audiologists. However, hearing function is an important outcome and recreational therapists should be familiar with the impact that hearing loss has on clients and how individuals with physical disabilities locate sound.

Hearing loss (b230) can have a significant impact on individuals with disabilities and how they function in their environment. The Hearing Handicap Inventory for the Elderly Screening Version (HHIE-S) (Ventry & Weinstein, 1983) is a 10-item questionnaire developed to assess how an individual perceives the social and emotional effects of hearing loss. The higher the HHIE-S score, the greater the handicapping effect of a hearing impairment. Possible scores range from 0 (no handicap) to 40 (maximum handicap). Individuals should be referred to a hearing specialist for further assessment if the HHIE-S score is higher than 10 points.

Vestibular Functions (b235)

Vestibular function is "sensory functions of the inner ear related to position, balance and movement" (WHO, 2001, p. 65). Balance is typically impaired by the loss of function in one of the following three systems: sensory (e.g., vision, vestibular/semicircular ear canals, proprioception), skeletal/muscular (e.g., upper and lower extremities, trunk, neck), or central nervous system (e.g., reflexes, learned skills, synergistic actions). Because balance requires the integration of these three systems, most balance assessments require performing tasks that require sensory, skeletal, and central nervous system components. Recreational therapists should be concerned with the assessment of balance because many individuals with physical disabilities, including older adults and those with brain and spinal cord injuries, have balance deficiencies (Skalko et al., 2013).

Application of Balance to Individuals With Disabling Conditions   Balance is a critical function that is impacted by neurological capacities within many populations served by the recreational therapist. For example, patients with spinal cord injuries (SCI) often have balance deficits because of lost or reduced muscle function resulting from the inability of the brain to transmit motor neuron impulses (Torhaug, Brurok, Hoff, Helgerudand, & Leivseth, 2016). Because a spinal cord injury often affects those systems required for balance (i.e., sensory, skeletal muscular, and central nervous system), balance deficiencies remain a critical focus within the scope of RT practice when working with individuals with SCI (Skalko et al., 2013). A variability in balance would be evident when an individual sustains a cervical- or thoracic-level SCI and neurological function is affected within the neck and torso region. An individual with a full neurological loss of function typically loses balance below the affected spinal column. For example, an individual with a C7 (i.e., seventh cervical vertebrae) quadriplegia injury would typically have balance issues that would start in the torso region and higher, because those motor areas are served by the cervical region of the spinal column. Conversely, the individual with a T12 (i.e., twelfth thoracic vertebrae) paraplegia would have relatively good balance because the region of the spinal column that serves the torso region would be unaffected. A higher injury level on the spinal column tends to have a greater impact on an individual's balance because of the significant loss of motor, sensation, and central nervous function. The recreational therapist should select balance assessments that fit their client's functional abilities. For example, many balance assessments require the individual to ambulate. Therefore, for the individual unable to ambulate, the recreational therapist should incorporate balance assessments that can be completed from a seated position.

Balance Theory

The complexities within balance make it a difficult construct to assess (Huxham, Goldie,

& Patla, 2001). Huxham and colleagues (2001) suggested that balance is a product of task and the environment in which an individual performs the task. They further suggested that there are certain biomechanical (physical) and information-processing (cognitive) aspects required of balance control and therefore there should be multifaceted approaches to balance assessment.

Before the many ways to assess balance are presented, conceptual definitions integral to an understanding of balance should be examined. First, balance tasks are different within motion and motionless environments because the amount of information processing and reactive biomechanical tasks increase as the balance-control task is increased. Therefore, when one is in a motionless position, the individual is said to be using *static balance* to maintain postural stability (Kamoun, Yahia, Ksentini, Ghroubi, & Elleuch, 2017). More specifically, *postural stability* is defined as the maintenance of an upright posture during quiet stance (Kamoun et al., 2017). Conversely, the ability of the body to maintain the balance point while in motion is known as *dynamic balance* (Kamoun et al., 2017). Because the task of maintaining balance while in motion is different and more challenging than while not in motion, it is important to differentiate the two and examine the biomechanical tasks within each situation.

Biomechanics of Balance Assessment

Because balance requires multiple interaction of human systems, assessment requires an approach that incorporates multidimensional perspectives. The following approaches to balance measurement focus on the biomechanics or physical task of balancing.

Timed Up and Go Test (TUG)   The TUG (Podsiadlo & Richardson, 1991) is a simple test that measures, in seconds, the time taken by an individual to stand up from a standard chair (approximate seat height of 46 cm, arm height 65 cm), walk a distance of three meters (approximately 10 feet), turn, walk back to the chair, and sit down. The client wears their regular footwear and uses their customary walking aid (none, cane, walker). On the word *go* they are to get up and walk at a comfortable and safe pace to a line on the floor three meters away, turn, return to the chair, and sit down again. The client walks through the test once before being timed in order to become familiar with the test. No physical assistance is given by the recreational therapist. Either a stopwatch or a wristwatch with a second hand can be used to time the trial. There is no time limit for the test and the client can stop and rest if needed. Once the TUG time has been established, the therapist can use it as a baseline or compare to normative scores for age (Bischoff, Stahelin, Monsch, Iverson, Weyh, von Dechend, et al., 2003) and fall prediction (Boulgarides, McGinty, Willett, & Barnes, 2003).

Functional Reach Test (FRT) and Multidirectional Reach Test (MDRT)   The ability to reach is an excellent task to assess balance and is commonly integrated in many tests because it incorporates biomechanics, postural control, and proprioceptive feedback. The FRT (Duncan, Weiner, Chandler, & Studenski, 1990) and MDRT (Newton, 2001) are simple tests that measure balance by assessing the maximum distance an individual can reach without stepping or losing balance. Prior to measurement, the recreational therapist should mount a yardstick on a wall at shoulder height. A measurement tool can also be constructed to assist in data collection by using PVC piping securely positioned on a wall using tape and placed at the level of the participants' shoulder horizontal to the floor. The client is then asked to position themselves close to but not touching the wall or measuring stick with their arm outstretched and hand unfisted. The recreational therapist notes the starting position by determining what number the end of the middle finger lines up with on the yardstick. The client should reach as far forward as they can without taking a step, keeping their feet flat on the floor and their hand at the level of the ruler. The recreational therapist then records the end position of the knuckles on the middle finger lines against the ruler. The difference between the starting and ending position numbers represents the distance reached. If the client moves their feet, that trial should be discarded and the attempt should be repeated. Guard the client during the task to prevent a fall. Clients are given two practice trials, then their performance on an additional three trials is recorded and averaged. This protocol represents the Functional Reach Test (FRT).

The MDRT includes the same protocol but continues by asking participants to reach backward (backward reach), left (lateral reach left), and right (lateral reach right) for three trials in each direction in the same manner. Location of the tip of the middle finger is recorded in inches at the starting and ending positions of each trial and the "trial distance" (inches) is obtained by determining the difference between the two position numbers (Newton, 2001). Participants are given the option of completing one practice trial to ensure adequate comprehension of instructions followed by three recorded test trials. The average of all three test trials for each direction is recorded as the total distance reached. If the participant's feet move during any trial, then that trial is discarded. For measures of forward reach, participants are given the opportunity of choosing to use either their right or left arm but are required to stay consistent throughout the test.

Modified Functional Reach Test (mFRT)

The FRT and the MDRT both require the individual to be able to stand for completion. If a client is unable to stand, the recreational therapist should consider the mFRT. The mFRT is similar to the FRT and MDRT except that the client is seated with hips, knees, and ankles positioned at 90 degrees of flexion with feet positioned flat on the floor. If the client is able to use his or her lower extremities to assist in balance, they are asked to suspend their feet above the ground during the test so their lower extremities do not assist in the reaching task.

If a client has an affected side, they are also asked to sit with the unaffected side near the wall/measuring device and lean forward for testing. Clients are allowed to sit and rest for 15 seconds between trials. The mFRT has been found to reliably measure balance in physical disability populations including those with spinal cord injury (Lynch, Leahy, & Barker, 1998) and stroke (Katz-Leurer, Fisher, Neeb, Schwartz, & Carmeli, 2009).

Cognitive Aspects of Balance

Another dimension of balance for many individuals with physical disabilities is related to cognitive aspects of balance, specifically one's confidence, or fall efficacy, with performing a task that requires balance. Skalko and colleagues (2013) suggested that measuring fall efficacy is important as it reflects how confident an individual may feel about their functional ability to balance. It is important for the recreational therapists to understand balance and perceived ability in order to prevent falls within physical disability populations.

Activities-Specific Balance Confidence Test (ABC Scale)

The ABC Scale (Powell & Myers, 1995) is a valid and reliable 16-item survey used to measure fall efficacy. It has commonly been used with older adults to measure an individual's confidence in performing tasks requiring balance (Skalko et al., 2013). During the ABC Scale, clients are asked to rate on a Likert scale their confidence (fall efficacy) of when they felt they would lose their balance or become unsteady in the course of performing certain daily activities. Scores are then established by taking an average of the individual's total responses (total ABC score divided by 16 = % of self-confidence). Higher scores on the ABC Scale indicate the client has higher confidence in their balance abilities.

Sensation of Pain (b280)

Pain is defined as "sensation of unpleasant feeling indicating potential or actual damage to some body structure" (WHO, 2001, p. 68). The ICF provides multiple pain classification codes based on the location of the pain source. The International Association for the Study of Pain (1994) identifies the four most common types of pain: low back pain (27%), severe headache or migraine pain (15%), neck pain (15%), and facial ache or pain (4%). In 1984, the International Association for the Study of Pain (IASP) established a system for assessing and describing chronic pain better by recommending that pain be classified according to the following specific characteristics:

a. region of the body involved (e.g., upper arm, head),

b. system that may be causing the pain (e.g., nervous),

c. duration,

d. intensity and time since onset, and

e. potential cause.

Because pain is determined by one's perception and tolerance, self-report is the most valid way to assess pain (Amico, 2016).

Numerical Pain Scales

The easiest and most common way to assess pain is to ask the client to self-report the intensity of the pain. There are many versions of self-reported numerical pain scales that could be used to assess a client's current state or a pre-post measurement to indicate change in pain status. For example, the 0-10 Pain Scale asks the client: "On a scale of 1-10, with 0 being 'no pain' and 10 being 'the most severe pain ever experienced,' what is your current level of pain?"

Visual Analog Scales (VAS)

Others have suggested the use of a Visual Analog Scale to measure pain intensity (Turk & Melzack, 2001). The VAS is another way of assessing pain intensity by using a more quantitative approach with more deviation beyond the typical Likert anchors (i.e., no pain, moderate pain, severe pain). The VAS (see figure 7.1) uses a horizontal line with word anchors at the extremes. The client is allowed to mark along the line (10 cm long) to represent the degree of pain intensity. The recreational therapist then measures distance of mark indicated. This measurement can be more exact than a simple Likert scale and can measure current pain state or used as pre-post measurement to assess pain change.

Pain Faces Scales

Instead of numbers, others have developed image scales, or Pain Faces Scales, that represent facial expressions of pain (Wong & Baker, 1988). Pain Faces Scales have been particularly helpful for populations that have difficulty cognitively assessing pain such as children, individuals with language barriers, and individuals with cognitive barriers (Wong & Baker, 1988). The Wong-Baker FACES Pain Rating Scale was designed specifically for assessing pain in children over the age of three and has been found to be valid in assessing pain in pediatric populations (Wong & Baker, 1988).

Jaywant and Pai (2003-04) provided some evidence of reliability and rating accuracy when they found that the pain ratings by burn patients using the Visual Analog Scale (VAS), Pain Faces Scale (PFS), and Numerical Pain Scale (NPS) all were highly correlated with one another. Pain remains an important outcome to measure and treat in recreational therapy practice with clients with physically disabling conditions (ATRA, 2019).

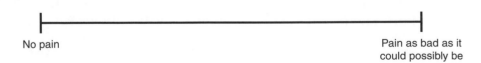

No pain

Pain as bad as it could possibly be

FIGURE 7.1   Visual Analog Scale (VAS) for pain assessment.

Based on I. Thong et al., "The Validity of Pain Intensity Measures: What Do the NRS, VAS, VRS, and FPS-R Measure?" *Scandinavian Journal of Pain* 18, no 1 (2018): 99-107.

Cardiovascular Systems

The human cardiovascular system consists of the heart, blood vessels, and the blood that the blood vessels transport. The recreational therapist works with many individuals with cardiovascular issues, including stroke patients, cardiac rehab patients, or individuals who may be obese or require physical training. Testing and monitoring cardiac outcomes is important for the recreational therapist to

a. assess patient safety before, during, and after various treatment programs involving exercise,

b. determine target outcome goals, and

c. obtain support for evidence-based treatment for RT interventions.

While the appropriateness of RT for a client is always determined by a physician, it is even more critical for the recreational therapist to know how to monitor cardiac outcomes in all individuals with physical disabilities.

Heart Functions (b410)

Heart function is "functions of pumping the blood in adequate or required amounts and pressure throughout the body" (WHO, 2001, p. 74). ICF classification of heart function includes all cardiac functions, including heart rate and blood pressure. Each year, more than 350,000 Americans have a cardiac arrest and only about one in 10 survives (AHA, 2017). Measuring and monitoring these cardiac outcomes can be important for recreational therapists to ensure client safety and track functional goals.

Heart Rate (b4100) Measurement   Heart rate is "function related to the number of times the heart contracts every minute" (WHO, 2001, p. 74). All individuals have different heart rates and even heart rates change over one's lifetime due to a variety of genetic and biological factors. The general idea is that heart rate indicates how hard the heart must work to adequately provide blood to the body. The lower the heart rate, the less the heart has to work. The human heart has a maximal capacity of 220 beats per minute, but no one should ever come close to that figure, because it will result in cardiac failure. That is why therapists and trainers commonly help clients calculate their estimated submaximal target heart range suggesting individuals do not exceed 80 percent ([220 – age] × .80). It is generally thought that those in better physical shape have lower heart rates as a result of their physical conditioning (ACSM, 2017). There are many ways to assess heart rates in clients. The most common way to measure heart rate is to test one's pulse (AHA, 2017). Therapists or clients themselves can measure pulse with the following steps:

1. Locate the pulse at either the carotid (on the neck just to the right side of the windpipe) or radial (backside of the wrist near thumb side) artery.

2. Using the tips of the first two fingers (not the thumb), press *lightly* over the blood vessels on the wrist or neck.

3. Count the number of pulses for 10 seconds and multiply by six to find beats per minute.

This number represents *resting heart rate*. The normal range for adults is 60 to 100 beats per minute (AHA, 2017). Although there is certainly a relationship between heart rate and blood pressure, they are two separate measurements and indicators of health (AHA, 2017).

Blood Pressure (BP) (b420) Measurement
BP is a "function of maintaining the pressure of blood within the arteries" (WHO, 2001, p. 76). More specifically, BP is an indicator of the force of blood moving though the blood vessels. A rising heart rate does not necessarily cause one's blood pressure to increase at the same rate (AHA, 2017). Even though an individual's heart is beating more times per minute, healthy blood vessels dilate (get larger) to allow more blood to flow. High blood pressure

(HBP), or *hypertension*, means the pressure in your arteries is higher than it should be. According to the American Heart Association (2017), about 80 million Americans over age 20, or one in three adults, have hypertension and may not even know it. Persistent hypertension can lead to certain health conditions including cerebrovascular accident (stroke), hypertensive nephropathy (chronic renal failure), or myocardial infarction (heart attack). BP is indicated as two important numbers measured in mm, including *systolic* (the top number) and *diastolic* (bottom number). The systolic number represents the pressure during a heart contraction and therefore is the higher of the two numbers. The diastolic number represents the pressure when the heart is relaxed, or between beats, and is the lower of the two numbers. According to the AHA (2017), normal blood pressure is below 120/80 mmHg. An adult individual is said to be in prehypertension when their systolic pressure is 120 to 139 or diastolic pressure is 80 to 89, or when both levels are in the higher range. Hypertension, or HBP, is a pressure of 140 systolic or higher and/or 90 diastolic or higher that stays high over a consistent period of time.

To measure BP, one needs a stethoscope and a sphygmomanometer (i.e., blood pressure cuff). Blood pressure cuffs come in various pediatric and adult sizes and should fit appropriately on the upper arm. A good general rule for fit is the 80 percent rule that suggests that a cuff should cover 80 percent of one's upper arm. The blood pressure measurement technique is as follows:

1. Make sure the round end of the stethoscope is placed under the blood pressure cuff.

2. Inflate the sphygmomanometer (blood pressure cuff) to a little above 180 mmHg. This collapses the major arteries to the arm (this may be somewhat uncomfortable).

3. Slowly release air by gently turning the air valve and watch the pressure drop (3 mmHg per second).

4. Listen for the first sound you hear; this will be the systolic blood pressure. The sound is the blood now flowing in the artery, which means that the systolic pressure is now greater than the pressure in the blood pressure cuff.

5. As the pressure continues to drop, the sound will at some point no longer be heard—this will be the diastolic blood pressure measurement.

The recreational therapist should take the resting heart rate and blood pressure of clients with physical disabilities before beginning programs requiring physical exertion. The recreational therapist can use the readings to establish a baseline for target heart ranges for therapeutic change, as well as compare to American Heart Association (AHA) prehypertensive readings for further precautions suggested by the participant's physician.

Respiration Functions (b440)

Another important function of the cardiovascular system involves functions of inhaling air into the lungs, facilitating the exchange of gases between the oxygen and blood (WHO, 2001). The measurement of these functions is certainly well beyond the scope and training of recreational therapists. However, recreational therapists often use exercise and physical activities for clients to involve and even extend their respiratory and cardiovascular capacities and therefore should be aware of techniques used to monitor exercise intensities.

Exercise Tolerance (b455)　Exercise tolerance is "functions related to respiratory and cardiovascular capacity as required for enduring physical exertion" (WHO, 2001, p. 80). Again, therapists programming exercise and physical activity for individuals with physical disabilities should be familiar with methods to assess the intensity of one's physical exertion in order to maintain safe levels and track treatment progress.

Borg Rating of Perceived Exertion 6-20 (RPE 6-20)

Borg RPE 6-20 (Borg, 1998) is a common method used to assess an individual's perceived level of exertion during a physical activity. It is based on the physical sensations a person experiences during physical activity, including increased heart rate, increased respiration or breathing rate, increased sweating, and muscle fatigue. The scale ranges from 6 (no exertion at all) to 20 (maximal exertion). The Borg RPE 6-20 is a subjective measure, but a person's exertion rating has been demonstrated to provide a good estimate of the actual heart rate during physical activity (Borg, 1998). Borg (1998) found that an estimated heart rate can be calculated by multiplying the RPE 6-20 rating by 10. For example, if the individual rates his or her physical exertion as 13, multiplying the rating by 10 equals 130 bpm (beats per minute). The recreational therapist can use the RPE 6-20 to assess a client's exercise tolerance and/or intensity during physical activity.

Arm Ergometer Test

The Arm Ergometer Test has been used to assess exercise tolerance in individuals with physical disabilities (Pollock, Miller, Linnerud, Laughridge, Coleman, & Alexander, 1974). The arm ergometer is an exercise device that requires the participant to move the handles in a circular motion to generate one's full aerobic capacity through one-minute maximal effort intervals. Because some individuals with physical disabilities have limited to no function in lower extremities, the arm ergometer is useful in assessing exercise tolerance and aerobic capacity. The recreational therapist can use the Arm Ergometer Test to assess one's baseline exercise tolerance and a comparative level for treatment progress. Sawka, Foley, Pimental, Toner, and Pandolf (1982) provided arm crank protocols and normative values for individuals with physical disabilities.

Six-Minute Walk Test (6MWT)

The 6MWT is a timed distance walk test developed by Balke (1963) and was initially developed to assess exercise capacity and functional status in persons with cardiorespiratory disorders. However, it has recently become one of the most widely applied assessments of exercise capacity and functional capacity (Rikli & Jones, 1998). The test could not be any simpler to perform—it only requires the patient to walk as far as they possibly can in six minutes. The primary outcome measured is the total distance walked in the time period allotted. While the test was initially developed for cardiac rehabilitation patients, it has become a functional fitness test of older adults who use orthopedic devices when walking, as well as people who have difficulty balancing.

Six-Minute Push Test (6MPT)

The 6MPT is an adaptation of the 6MWT for wheelchair users. The 6MPT is a maximal test of aerobic capacity and has been found valid and reliable in persons with spinal cord injuries above T10 (Cowan, Callahan, & Nash, 2012). The following supplies are needed for this test: cones, tape measure, stopwatch, floor tape, and a heart rate monitor. Prior to the test, the recreational therapist should use the cones and floor tape to create the course with a two-way loop that measures 15 meters (or 49.21 feet) each way so it creates a 30-meter loop. The client's pretest resting heart rate (RHR) should be recorded. The recreational therapist should then instruct the client that they are to push back and forth in the loop for six minutes straight. The client can rest periodically during the test but needs to resume as soon as possible to push as far as possible for six minutes. The recreational therapist will keep track of how many laps the client completes. When time expires, the recreational therapist will mark the location of the client with a piece of floor tape, immediately record the client's heart rate and the number of laps completed, and measure the additional distance after the final lap (the number of meters/feet in the final partial lap) to calculate the total distance pushed. Total distance pushed is then compared to norms established by Cowan and colleagues (2012) to determine "low," "medium," and "high" fitness levels. The 6MPT has been demonstrated to be as effective as the Arm Ergometer Test in reaching peak levels of oxygen consumption (Cowan et al., 2012).

Neuromusculoskeletal and Movement-Related Functions

Neuromuscular function is often impaired as a result of physical disability (WHO, 2017). The recreational therapist working with individuals with physical disabilities requires knowledge of neuromuscular and movement-related functions and those instruments commonly used to measure these outcomes. This section will address functions related to mobility of joint (flexibility), muscle power, and muscle endurance.

Mobility of Joint (b710)

Mobility of joint is the "functions of the range and ease of movement of a joint" (WHO, 2001, p. 94) and is traditionally called *flexibility* or *range of motion* (ROM). Flexibility is an important functional outcome for individuals with physical disabilities, because it is integral to many life skills such as pushing a wheelchair, ambulation, dressing, and performing recreation skills (WHO, 2017). Shoulders, hamstrings, and trunk muscles are the most common muscles tested for flexibility in individuals with mobility impairments (NCHPAD, 2017).

Goniometer   Range of motion is measured in degrees of movement (0-360) and is most commonly measured using a device called a *goniometer* (see figure 7.2). Goniometer can literally be translated as *gonia*, which means "angle," and *meter*, which means "measure."

All joints have a normal range of motion in relation to the "neutral" or zero starting point (Burlingame & Blaschko, 2010). The goniometer is commonly used for objective measurements in order to accurately track progress in rehabilitation programs. The goniometer is more commonly used by other allied health providers such as physical therapists and athletic trainers, but the recreational therapist should be familiar with normal ROM standards for program planning. While the goniometer is

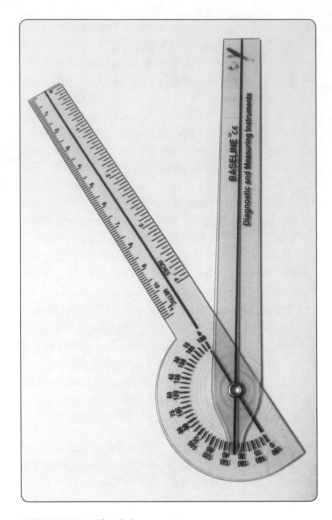

FIGURE 7.2   Flexibility goniometer.

the most common way to assess flexibility, there are multiple performance tests that can provide ROM assessment and screening for recreational therapists.

YMCA/Sit and Reach Test   The YMCA/Sit and Reach Test (Wells & Dillon, 1952) is one of the oldest and most common tests for back and leg flexibility. It is appropriate for individuals with the ability to sit unassisted because it requires the use of a "sit and reach box" that measures how far one can reach in a seated position on the floor. Before performing the test, the client should do a general warm-up and stretch for 5 to 10 minutes. A client should never perform the test without warming up their muscle groups. The recreational therapist should place the sit and reach box against a wall or immovable backstop. The client is then instructed to remove his or her shoes and sit on the floor facing the box with a straight back and legs fully extended so that the knees are not in a locked position. The client's feet are against the sit and reach box at shoulder-width apart. The client is then asked to flex at the waist, extend their arms forward with palms facing down one over the other, and reach as far as possible without bouncing and jerking in order to push the measurement arm on the sit and reach box. The client should hold this position for three seconds. The test should be completed three times with the best of the three trials recorded to the nearest half-inch. Results are then compared to normative scores for the client's age and gender (ACSM, 2017).

Back Scratch Test   The Back Scratch Test (Rikli & Jones, 2001), one of many tests included in the Senior Fitness Test developed by Rikli and Jones (2001), can also be used with individuals with physical disabilities (NCHPAD, 2017). Because it was developed for older adults, the norms were established for only that population comparison (Rikli & Jones, 2013), but the test remains an adequate test for assessing upper body (shoulder joint) flexibility, which is particularly important for wheelchair users (NCHPAD, 2017). The only equipment needed for this test is a ruler/tape measure to record best results to the nearest half-inch. The client begins by reaching with his or her preferred hand with palm down and fingers extended over the shoulder and down the back while reaching with the other hand, palm up and fingers extended, toward the first hand. The client should be allowed to choose the best or preferred hand throughout the trial period to promote his or her best attempt. The recreational therapist should administer two practice trials and two test trials. The ruler is then used to measure the finger overlap (positive score) or gap (negative score) between the middle fingers of each hand. If the fingers just touch each other, the recreational therapist should record the score as a zero. Therefore, a higher score would

be indicative of greater shoulder ROM. This measure can be beneficial to the recreational therapist when measuring a change in a client's ROM from baseline.

Muscle Power (b730)

The ICF defines muscle power as "functions related to the force generated by the contraction of a muscle or muscle groups" (WHO, 2001, p. 96). Muscle power is an important functional outcome for individuals with physically disabling conditions. Individuals with physical disabilities require significant muscle strength to perform life activities and functional skills (Stumbo & Peterson, 2009). Unfortunately, many physical disabilities such as spinal cord injury, Parkinson's disease, multiple sclerosis, muscular dystrophy, and amyotrophic lateral sclerosis (ALS) result in deteriorating or even complete loss of muscle power. Therefore, it is critical to measure and subsequently treat individuals with physical disabilities who have deficiencies in muscular power in order to provide opportunities to promote full and meaningful lives.

One-Repetition Maximum Test (1-RM)   The 1-RM test is considered the gold standard for assessing muscle strength in nonlaboratory situations (Macht, Abel, Mullineaux, & Yates, 2016). 1-RM is the maximum amount of weight one is able to lift in one attempt. This test should follow the American College of Sports Medicine's (ACSM, 2017) protocols with adaptations and modifications depending on the client's functional level and ability. While the 1-RM can be used with many lifts, one of the most common and easiest for individuals with physical disabilities is the upper extremity chest press. An exercise bench, bench press bar, and assorted weighted plates are required for this test. Because the test requires the client to bench press their *maximal* amount of weight, it is important to gradually build to this lift to avoid injury. The client should warm up by completing five to 10 submaximal repetitions using the bench press. Following the first warm-up, the client should rest for one minute before they perform two more warm-up sets of two to five repetitions at light to moderate weight with a two-minute rest between sets. Following the warm-up, the sets will be a single repetition as the weight approaches the client's maximum amount of weight. The recreational therapist should allow for three to five minutes of rest between trials. The 1-RM final weight lifted should be accomplished within four attempts; anything more will invalidate the maximum amount due to fatigue. Determining the starting resistance can be difficult and requires observation of the client's lifts during the warm-up period. The ACSM protocol suggests that the weight should be progressively increased during the trials by 2.5 to 20 kilograms (5.5 to 44 pounds). While the ACSM (2017) provides strength categories for upper body strength based on the 1-RM Test, they might not be applicable to individuals with physical disabilities. Therefore, scores should be used as a baseline value to track changes and improvements in muscular strength.

Multiple RM/Predicted 1-RM Test

Research has indicated that injuries may be associated with performing a 1-RM test in some populations and the use of a means to estimate or predict a 1-RM may be more appropriate (Macht et al., 2016). If the client is new to exercise, deconditioned, a senior adult, or for any other reason the 1-RM Test is not suitable, the recreational therapist should select a Multiple RM/Predicted 1-RM test. This method is a modification of the 1-RM in which an individual performs multiple repetitions at a specified submaximal weight load and those results are entered into an equation to *predict* one's 1-RM amount. This method is often seen as a safer way to determine one's strength for those populations that may not be appropriate for a 1-RM test (Macht et al., 2016). The Multiple RM/Predicted 1-RM test can still establish a baseline for the client's muscular strength based on the number of repetitions performed with submaximal loads (Niewiadomski, Laskowska, Gasiorowska, Cybulski, Strasz, & Langfor, 2008). Niewiadomski and colleagues (2008) suggested this method is safer to avoid cardiovascular risks

and muscle soreness. The warm-up protocol is the same for the Multiple RM/Predicted 1-RM test, but the individual stops well below their maximal weight. Once they reach a comfortable weight lifted, a formula is used to predict the 1-RM amount. While there are many formulas used to predict 1-RM (ACSM, 2017), the Brzycki Predicted 1-RM Formula (1993) has been found to be highly correlated with actual 1-RM scores (do Nascimento, Cyrino, Nakamura, Romanzini, Pianca, & Queiroga, 2007). The Brzycki Predicted 1-RM Formula is:

$$\text{Predicted 1-RM} = W \times (36 / (37 - R));$$
$$(R = \text{reps}, W = \text{weight})$$

The recreational therapist inputs the amount of weight lifted and repetitions performed into the formula to calculate the predicted 1-RM.

Medicine Ball Throw Test

The Medicine Ball Throw Test (NCHPAD, 2017) is a test of upper extremity strength requiring the individual to throw a medicine ball as far as possible while seated or standing. To administer, a measuring tape, medicine ball (various weights), and masking tape is needed. This test does not have normative standards for comparative interpretation. Therefore, the weight of the medicine ball can be varied depending on client strength and further used to assess, measure, and track progress with upper extremity strength during treatment programs. While the client is seated or standing, the recreational therapist should ask the client to throw the medicine ball as far as possible in a forward direction as an overhead or chest pass. To maintain consistency in tracking progress, the therapist should always retest with the same weight and throwing technique during each phase of the measurement. For measurement accuracy, the recreational therapist should put masking tape where the medicine ball first hit the ground, not where it rolls. Measurement of the distance from the client to the masking tape mark represents the baseline for upper extremity strength. The same procedure can be used following a strength regimen to measure progress. Because there are relationships between how much one can lift to how *long* one can perform (ACSM, 2017), it is also important to assess muscular endurance in individuals with physical disabilities.

Muscle Endurance (b740)

Muscular endurance is defined as "functions related to sustaining muscle contraction for the required period of time" (WHO, 2001, p. 98). Muscular endurance is another neuromuscular outcome important to individuals with physical disabilities. For example, individuals who use wheelchairs must typically use their arms to propel themselves. Compared with the legs, arm function is far less efficient in promoting mobility and typically results in lower physical capacity and consequential limited muscular endurance (Torhaug et al., 2016). Therefore, it is critical for the RT professional and other therapists to assess muscular endurance to determine treatment interventions that promote the development of muscular endurance (Torhaug et al., 2016).

Push-Up Endurance Test   The Push-Up Endurance Test (Pescatello & American College of Sports Medicine, 2014) assesses muscular endurance by seeing how many push-ups an individual can do. A floor mat can be used for this test. For men, hands should be pointing forward and under the shoulders with head up; for women, hands should be shoulder-width apart with head up. The recreational therapist should consider performing a proper push-up to ensure clients understand the proper push-up technique. The client must raise their body by straightening the elbows and then lowering the body to return to the down position without allowing his or her stomach to touch the floor. The score is determined by the maximal number of push-ups performed consecutively without rest in between attempts. The test is stopped once the client strains forcibly or is unable to maintain the appropriate push-up technique within two repetitions. The client's number of push-ups can then be compared to standards of comparison of age and gender (ACSM, 2017). If the client is unable to perform a push-up, the test can be adapted so the client performs a plank (holding the push-up position without moving) until they are unable to hold the position. Although this may be an adequate way to monitor progress over time, comparing results to established standards cannot be used because the plank protocol is different.

Curl-Up/Sit-Up Test   This test, also adapted from Pescatello and ACSM (2014), is an assessment of abdominal muscular endurance for individuals with physical disabilities that counts the maximum number of curl-up (i.e., abdominal crunches) repetitions performed. To administer the test, tape, a tape measure, and a metronome will be needed. If the client has limited abdominal or core function, a counterweight such as resistance bands, dumbbells, and plates may also be needed to complete the curl-up movement. The therapist can also allow the client to complete the maximum number of curl-ups at their own pace, without using the metronome. NCHPAD (2017) recommends that if the client is less than 45 years old, the therapist can place two strips of tape on the floor 12 centimeters apart; if they are over 45, place tape eight centimeters apart. Clients can then lie down on their back, with their arms at their sides, so their fingertips touch the first strip. A wedge can also be placed under the client's legs to help bend their knees approximately 90 degrees. To reach the top position, the client will sit up and reach their fingers forward until they touch the second piece of tape. The recreational therapist should set a metronome to 40 beats per minute to help maintain a consistent pace. On the first beep, the client will curl up to the top position and then return to the bottom position on the second beep and continue that pattern. A repetition is counted every time the client returns to the starting position. The test is stopped when 75 curl-ups are achieved or the client is unable to maintain the beat. If the client is unable to transfer onto a mat or the ground, a cable machine can be used to perform the abdominal crunches. The therapist may adjust the resistance to a light setting to provide a counterweight if needed. The client will complete as many of these curl-ups as possible. While this test is without specific standardized protocols and does not have normative standards, it can be used to track progress for clients needing to improve abdominal endurance.

Measurement of Activities and Participation

The ICF includes functions that are covered in a range of areas of social and community life. *Activities* are defined as the "execution of a task or action as an individual" (WHO, 2001, p. 123). *Participation* is defined as "the involvement in a life situation" (p. 123). This section of the ICF is particularly important to recreational therapists working with individuals with physical disabilities because it directly relates to those tasks and recreation and life activity situations. While there are many activities and participation functions to discuss, this section will examine those most important and relevant to RT practice, including mobility and community, social, and civic life.

Mobility

Mobility is an important issue for individuals with physical disabilities (WHO, 2017). Mobility is far beyond just moving—the ICF includes changing body positions, transferring from one place to another, carrying or manipulating objects, and walking. This section of the chapter will examine two commonly treated ICF mobility functions in individuals with physical disabilities, fine hand use and wheelchair mobility.

Fine Hand Use (d440)

Fine hand use is "performing the coordinated actions of handling objects, picking up, manipulating and releasing them using one's hand, fingers and thumb, such as required to lift coins off a table or turn a dial or knob" (WHO, 2001, p.142). The ICF further classifies hand function into areas including picking up (d4400), grasping (d4401), manipulating (d4402), and releasing (d4403). According to the U.S. Census Bureau (2010), about 19.9 million people have physical disabilities that make it difficult to do tasks like lifting or grasping. Therefore, many

allied health therapists measure and track hand function and it remains important for the recreational therapist to be aware of the terms and techniques used and to apply these to RT goals.

Measuring grip strength can be extremely useful in rehabilitation when establishing a baseline of strength, creating rehabilitation goals, and tracking improvements with strength training during rehabilitation (Petersen, Petrick, Connor, & Conklin, 1989). Nalebuff and Philips (1990) suggested that 20 pounds of hand grip strength is needed to perform most basic daily activities, but most therapists set higher goals to help clients achieve greater independence (Petersen et al., 1989). Grip strength has been considered so important that research has gone even further and suggested that hand grip strength can be an indicator of a client's *overall* strength (NCHPAD, 2017). Grip strength is commonly assessed with a device called a dynamometer to measure hand and finger grip strength (see figure 7.3).

When measuring hand grip strength, the therapist should be aware that grip strength can vary due to a number of factors such as gender, age, and dominant and nondominant hands (Bechtol, 1954). While Bechtol (1954) established the standard 10 percent rule that states that the dominant hand possesses a 10 percent greater grip strength than the nondominant hand, others have suggested the rule is valid for right-handed persons only (Petersen et al., 1989). While Mathiowetz, Weber, Volland, and Kashman (1984) suggested that certain dynamometers can use normative standards interchangeably, it is more appropriate for the recreational therapist to compare results with standards provided by the actual instrument used for testing. Sisto and Dyson-Hudson (2007) also suggested that certain types of dynamometers may be more appropriate for spinal cord injury clients due to limited neurological hand function and mechanical requirements of certain manufacturer brands.

Like all measurement performance tests, hand grip strength testing results can vary when different protocols are used. Therefore, established testing protocols should be used to

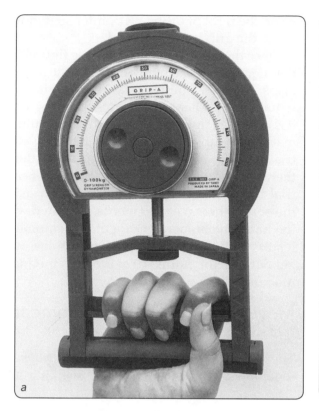
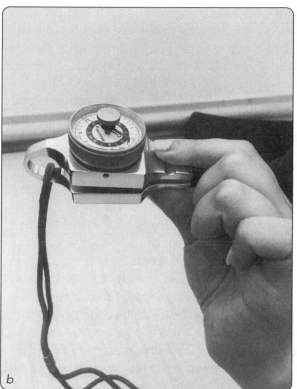

FIGURE 7.3   *(a)* Hand and *(b)* finger dynamometers.

maintain accuracy and duplication of results. For example, the dynamometer handle should ideally be adjusted to fit the client's hand—or if that's not possible, the handle should be set at the same setting for all clients. Also, the recreational therapist should perform multiple tests in order to get the best maximum score. Finally, hand grip strength test results can also be affected by the position of the wrist, elbow, and shoulder, so these should be standardized and adequate bracing or support should be used with individuals with physical conditions that require such support (NCHPAD, 2017).

The recreational therapist should conduct the hand dynamometer test by demonstrating the use of the instrument to the participant prior to testing. The protocol should include

a. standing, if able (individuals needing support should use adequate bracing),

b. placing arms at their sides not touching their body,

c. keeping elbow bent slightly, and

d. squeezing the dynamometer with as much force as possible, once for each measurement.

Three trials should be made with a pause of about 10 to 20 seconds between each trial to avoid the effects of muscle fatigue. The recreational therapist should record the result of each trial to the nearest pound or kilogram using the best of three measurements. Results should then be compared to age- and gender-specific norms provided by the dynamometer manufacturer.

Many fitness trainers and allied health therapists, including recreational therapists, may also be interested in finger grip strength, because it is needed to perform a range of activities requiring hand use. It is important for the recreational therapist to be familiar with measurement and interpretation of finger grip standards as they work with various physical disability populations. Like hand grip strength, finger grip strength is measured with a dynamometer (Mathiowetz et al., 1984) (see figure 7.3). Finger grip strength can be used to measure different types of grasping (d4401) and picking up grips (d4400) including a) *tip pinch* (e.g., thumb to index fingertip), b) *key pinch* (thumb pad to middle portion of index finger), and c) *Palmer pinch* (using thumb pad to pads of index and middle fingers) (see figure 7.4).

Finger pinch dynamometers are available from different manufacturers and models varying from two to 60 pounds of finger grip strength.

To administer the finger pinch grip test, the following procedures should be implemented. The gauge must be "zeroed" before each pinch test by setting the red maximum pointer and the black pointer at the zero marking. To do this, the therapist should rotate the small knob on top of the dial indicator in a counterclockwise direction until both are set to zero (see figure 7.5). Note that the red pointer arm must

be on the right of the black pointer so it moves when the grip test is initiated.

Once the gauge is set to zero (see figure 7.5), the client is asked to perform one of the desired grips. The red pointer (stationary arm) will remain at the client's maximum reading until it is reset (see figure 7.6). Three trials should be made with 10 to 20 seconds in between each trial to avoid muscle fatigue. The recreational therapist should then record the result of each trial to the nearest pound or kilogram using the best of three measurements. As stated with the hand dynamometer, finger dynamometer results should then be compared to age- and gender-specific norms provided by the manufacturer.

Moving Around Using Equipment (d465)

The ICF includes *moving around using equipment* (d465) as a function within the walking and

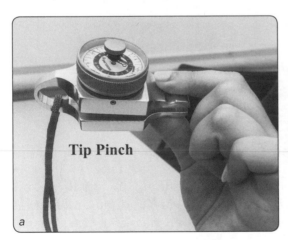

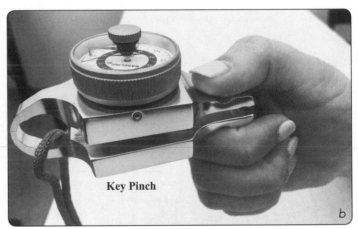

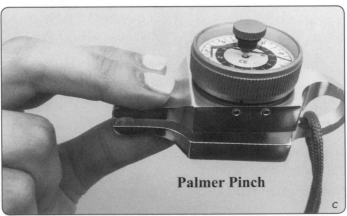

FIGURE 7.4 *(a)* Tip pinch, *(b)* key pinch, and *(c)* Palmer pinch finger grip positions.

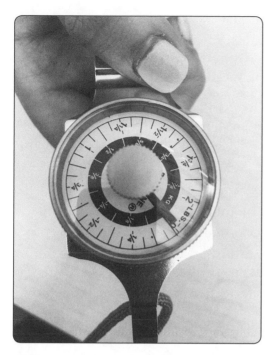

FIGURE 7.5   "Zeroing out" the finger pinch dynamometer.

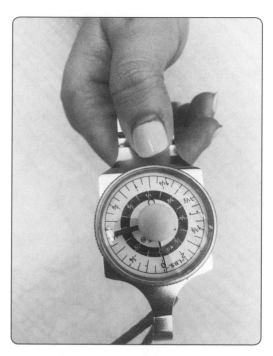

FIGURE 7.6   Finger pinch dynamometer stationary arm reading.

moving category. The ability of individuals with physical disabilities to use wheelchairs effectively for mobility is often directly related to their ability to function and live life more independently (WHO, 2017). The recreational therapist often includes wheelchair mobility as an outcome, particularly as it relates to community mobility, and therefore needs to include measures to assess and track progress (Burlingame & Blaschko, 2010).

Wheelchair Skills Test (WST)
The wheelchair mobility outcome measure for individuals with physical disabilities is typically defined as how safely and effectively a client can use a wheelchair in their own environment (Kirby, Swuste, Dupuis, MacLeod, & Monroe, 2002). However, the mobility challenges that face these individuals are immense and varied (WHO, 2017). The WST (Kirby et al., 2002) consists of 33 items that measure a client's functional wheelchair skills needed in daily life. The tasks involved begin with easier skills (e.g., braking, managing footrests) and progress to the more difficult skills (e.g., managing a 10 cm curb, wheelies). Each skill is scored by the therapist with a three-point ordinal scale where 0 is failure

to complete, 1 is partial completion, and 2 is for successful and safe completion. Higher scores on the WST reflect higher levels of wheelchair mobility independence. Sol and colleagues (2017) also developed an adapted version of the WST for pediatric wheelchair users.

Community, Social, and Civic Life

The utility of the ICF is the focus on the function of the individual with disabilities in a variety of settings. Another such area that is primary within the scope of RT practice is the inclusion of community, social, and civic life. This area is defined as "actions and tasks required to engage in organized social life outside the family, in community, social and civic areas of life" (WHO, 2001, p. 168). Many individuals with physical disabilities have difficulty engaging with their communities based on the many limitations as a result of their disability or existing constraints within society (WHO, 2017). Of all the ICF functional outcomes to address within physical disability, the recreational therapist may be positioned best to make an impact in recreation and leisure and community reintegration.

Recreation and Leisure (d920)

The ICF defines recreation and leisure as "engaging in any form of play, recreational or leisure activity, such as informal or organized play and sports, programs of physical fitness, relaxation, amusement or diversion, going to art galleries, museums, cinemas or theatres; engaging in crafts or hobbies, reading for enjoyment, playing musical instruments; sightseeing, tourism and travelling for pleasure" (WHO, 2001, p. 168). Recreational therapists are consistently required to measure the level of engagement within recreation activities. However, one historical issue in the measurement of recreation engagement is the overreliance of attendance data. The recreational therapist should understand the levels of recreation engagement, represented by the following:

- Attendance: A binary count of participants in a program or frequency of participation (e.g., "Was a client there or not?")

- Participation: A linear measurement of the quality of effort (e.g., "*How* did the client participate?" or "Were they 'harmful to others' or did they 'receive cathartic benefits'?")

- Involvement: The multifaceted dimension of one's cognitive and emotional engagement (e.g., "What did the activity *mean* to the client?")

Leisure Competence Measures (LCM)   The Functional Independence Measure (FIM) is the most widely accepted functional assessment measure in physical rehabilitation for individuals with physical disabilities. While it does incorporate many secondary outcomes important in recreation participation, it does not address competencies specific to successful recreation functioning (Kloseck, Crilly, & Hutchinson-Troyer, 2001). Therefore, the Leisure Competence Measure (LCM) (Kloseck & Crilly, 1997) was developed as a standardized tool that provides the recreational therapist with the ability to document current levels of functioning across eight recreation and leisure domains, including Leisure Awareness, Leisure Attitude, Leisure Skills, Cultural/Social Behaviors, Interpersonal Skills, Community Reintegration Skills, Social Contact, and Community Participation. Similar to the structure of the FIM, the LCM requires the recreational therapist to rate the client on a seven-point ordinal scale:

7: Complete independence

6: Modified independence

5: Modified dependence

4: Modified dependence with minimum assistance

3: Modified dependence with moderate assistance

2: Modified dependence with maximum assistance

1: Total dependence with total assistance

Kloseck and colleagues (2001) further evaluated the LCM and determined the instrument's sensitivity was such that it was able to detect changes in clients with different diagnoses. The LCM can be used to establish a baseline or track functional progress in the eight areas of recreation engagement.

Community Integration

Community integration (CI) is a primary duty and focus of RT services (ATRA, 2019). However, conceptualizing and measuring community reintegration remains a difficult task because of the different ways researchers and measurement experts define it and the multidimensional nature it possesses. For example, the ICF includes many different functional outcomes that are incorporated within CI, such as informal associations (d9100), confidence (d1266), problem solving (d1646), basic economic transactions (d860), mobility (e120), transportation (e540), recreation and leisure (d920), and relating with strangers (d730). While all of these ICF outcomes have some relationship to CI, there isn't one functional outcome in ICF representative of a single CI construct. Although the recreational therapist consistently provides CI outings and programs for clients with physical disabilities, it remains a difficult task to measure and track the impact of such programs without the use of consistent assessment protocols.

The Craig Handicap Assessment and Reporting Technique (CHART)

The CHART is a 27-item scale questionnaire designed to measure the level of community participation of individuals with spinal cord injuries (Whiteneck, Charlifue, Frankel, Fraser, Gardner, Gerhart, et al., 1992). It is divided into five categories: physical independence, mobility, social integration, economic self-sufficiency, and occupation. Each of the five subscales are transformed to a scale score ranging from 0 (complete handicap) to 100 (no handicap). Higher scores on the CHART represent higher levels of CI (maximum possible score is 500, indicating no handicap at all). The CHART assesses the extent of participation (handicap) for people living in the community, regardless of the number of years since their inpatient rehabilitation or involvement with the health care system.

The Community Integration Questionnaire (CIQ)

The CIQ was originally designed as a measurement of community integration for individuals with traumatic brain injury (Willer, Ottenbacher, & Coad, 1994). This 15-item test includes three subscales, which examine

a. home integration (e.g., Who does the grocery shopping at home? Who does the everyday housework?);

b. social integration (e.g., Who looks after your finances?); and

c. productive activities (e.g., Do you work or volunteer? How often?).

The CIQ has a total scale score range of 0 to 27, with possible ranges of 0 to 10 for the home subscale, 0 to 12 for the social subscale, and 0 to 5 for the productive subscale. Scores for these domains are generated based on the frequency of engaging in roles and activities, and responses are weighted according to level of independence in performing roles and activities. The CIQ has been validated for use with SCI populations (Gontkovsky, Russum, & Stokic, 2009), but some have suggested

the CIQ may be improved for use in SCI by including items that reflect higher levels of productive functioning, integration across the life span, and home- and Internet-based social functioning (Kratz, Chadd, Jensen, Kehn, & Kroll, 2015).

Finding Assessments for Measuring Physical Disability

Using the correct assessment instrument is critical to generating accurate results that assist the therapist in identifying outcomes that require treatment for individuals with physical disabilities (Stumbo & Peterson, 2009). While this chapter includes many different valid and reliable assessment instruments, it may be necessary for the RT to explore other options that meet the assessment needs of his or her participants with physical disabilities. The following resources are helpful in identifying and evaluating various instruments available to assess individuals with physical disabilities.

Rehabilitation Measures Database

The Rehabilitation Measures Database (RMD) (www.rehabmeasures.org) is a website developed by the Rehabilitation Institute of Chicago (RIC) and the Center for Rehabilitation Outcomes Research (CROR). Clinician reviewers provide a comprehensive review of assessments commonly used for rehabilitation. The database provides evidence-based summaries that include each instrument's psychometric properties, instructions for administration and scoring, and often a copy of the instrument for therapists to download or information about obtaining the instrument. The RMD has more than 300 instruments for use with a number of diagnoses, including stroke, spinal cord injury, and traumatic brain injury, among several others. The RMD is a valuable resource for the recreational therapist to search for and evaluate instruments to assess a variety of outcomes for individuals with physical disabilities.

Application of the Assessment Process With an Individual With a Physical Disability

Bill is a 26-year-old with C6 quadriplegia. He completed three months of physical rehabilitation and has been living in the community with his wife for the past nine months. Bill heard about the recreational therapist working in his community and met with her to gain more independence and become more active since his discharge. Sarah Bellinger, a CTRS working in Bill's community, agreed to meet with Bill to conduct an assessment. She asked Bill if he could access his inpatient rehabilitation records or have them transferred to her in order to provide some preliminary information. During the initial meeting, Sarah performed a battery of assessments. She used a recreation interest survey to assess Bill's preferred recreation and leisure (d920) activities, a hand and finger dynamometer test for fine hand use (d440), the WST for mobility (d498), the CHART for community reintegration, and the modified functional reach test for vestibular balance (b240). The information indicates Bill has had limited recreation engagement (d920) since his SCI but expressed interest in sports and exercise (d9201) with a desire to get stronger so that he can progress from his power chair to a manual wheelchair. He has expressed a small fear of going in the community by himself because he doesn't have confidence in his skills. Hand and finger dynamometer readings indicate below average fine hand use (d440), but appropriate considering his spinal cord injury level. The WST test indicated a score of 19 (out of 66) for mobility (d498) and the CHART scores ranged from 18 to 32 in all five areas of CI. Answer the following questions based on this information.

1. Discuss how the diagnosis of an SCI may have affected the CTRS's selection of assessment instruments.

2. What are some appropriate treatment goals based on the interpretation of the assessment performance data provided?

3. What are some preliminary interventions appropriate for Bill based on your interpretation of the assessment results?

National Center on Health, Physical Activity, and Disability (NCHPAD)

NCHPAD, founded in 1999, is a public health practice and resource center on health promotion for people with disabilities. NCHPAD seeks to help people with disabilities achieve health benefits through increased participation in all types of physical and social activities, including fitness and aquatic activities, recreational and sports programs, and adaptive equipment usage. NCHPAD provides resources for the recreational therapist, including articles, research, fitness assessment resources, and assessment implementation videos (www.nchpad.org/fitnesstesting) needed to help individuals with physical disabilities live active lives.

Summary

One of the most important aspects of the APIE (Assess, Plan, Implement, and Evaluate) process is skill of assessment (Burlingame & Blaschko, 2010). An *inaccurate* assessment of the client makes it impossible to program and implement effective interventions that successfully change the health outcomes of the client (Stumbo, 2009). Individuals with physical disabilities have a variety of diagnostic characteristics that require accurate and precise assessment in order to identify outcomes to treat effectively. This chapter has presented many of the physical attributes of this population and the respective strategies for valid and reliable assessment.

REFLECTION QUESTIONS

1. What role does assessment have when working with individuals with physical disabilities?
2. How does the physical disability itself affect the assessment of those clients with physical disabilities?
3. What are some factors that recreational therapists need to consider when choosing an assessment for individuals with physical disabilities?
4. Why would a recreational therapist need to know assessment information about individuals with physical disabilities even if they are not the primary team member responsible for the assessment?

REFERENCES

American College of Sports Medicine. (2017). *Guidelines for exercise testing and prescription* (10th ed.). Baltimore, MD: Lippincott, Williams & Wilkins.

American Heart Association. (2017). AHA News: New guidelines aim to prevent sudden cardiac death. Retrieved October 4, 2017, from www.heart.org/heartorg

American Therapeutic Recreation Association. (2019). About recreational therapy. Retrieved March 27, 2019, from https://www.atra-online.com/page/AboutRecTherapy

Amico, D. (2016). *Health & physical assessment in nursing.* Boston, MA: Pearson.

Azouvi, P., Bartolomea, P., Beis, J., Perennou, D., Pradat-Diehl, P., & Rousseaux, M. (2006). A battery of tests for the quantitative assessment of unilateral neglect. *Restorative Neurology and Neuroscience, 24,* 273-285.

Balke, B. (1963). *A simple field test for the assessment of physical fitness: Civil Aeromedical Research Institute Report.* Oklahoma City, OK: Federal Aviation Agency.

Bechtol, C.O. (1954). The use of a dynamometer with adjustable handle spacings. *The Journal of Bone and Joint Surgery, 36*(4), 820-832.

Bergego, C., Azouvi, P., Samuel, C., Marchal, F., Louis-Dreyfus, A., Jokic, C., et al. (1995). Validation d'une échelle d'evaluation fonctionnelle de l'heminegligence dans la vie quotidienne: L'echelle CB. *Annales de Réadaptation et de Médecine Physique, 38,* 183-189.

Bischoff, H.A., Stahelin, H.B., Monsch, A.U., Iverson, M.D., Weyh, A., von Dechend, M., et al. (2003). Identifying a cut-off point for normal mobility: A comparison study of the timed "up and go" test in community-dwelling and institutionalized elderly women. *Age and Ageing, 32,* 315-320.

Borg, G. (1998). *Borg's perceived exertion and pain scales.* Champaign, IL: Human Kinetics.

Boulgarides, L.K., McGinty, S.M., Willett, J.A, & Barnes, C.W. (2003). Use of clinical and impairment-based tests to predict falls by community-dwelling older adults. *Physical Therapy, 83*(4), 328-339.

Brzycki, M. (1993). Strength testing: Predicting a one-rep max from repetitions to fatigue. *Journal of Physical Education, Recreation, & Dance, 64,* 88-90.

Burlingame, J., & Blaschko, T.M. (2010). *Assessment tools for recreational therapy and related fields* (4th ed.). Ravensdale, WA: Idyll Arbor.

Chen, P., Hreha, K., Fotis, P., Goedert, K.M., & Barrett, A.M. (2012). Functional assessment of spatial neglect: A review of the Catherine Bergego scale and an introduction of the Kessler Foundation neglect assessment process. *Topics in Stroke Rehabilitation, 19*(5), 1423-1435.

Cowan, R.E., Callahan, M.K., & Nash, M.S. (2012). The 6-min push test is reliable and predicts low fitness in spinal cord injury. *Medicine & Science in Sports & Exercise, 44,* 1993-2000.

Duncan, P., Weiner, D., Chandler, J., & Studenski, S. (1990). Functional reach: A new clinical measure of balance. *Journal of Gerontology: Medical Sciences, 45,* M192-M197.

Eser, I., Durrie, D.S., Schwendeman, F., & Stahl, J.E. (2008). Association between ocular dominance and refraction. *Journal of Refractive Surgery, 24*(7), 685-689.

Gontkovsky, S.T., Russum, P., & Stokic, D.S. (2009). Comparison of the CIQ and chart short form in assessing community integration in individuals with chronic spinal cord injury: A pilot study. *Neurorehabilitation, 24*(2), 185-192.

Huxham, P., Goldie, P., & Patla, A.E. (2001). Theoretical considerations in balance assessment. *Australian Journal of Physiotherapy, 47*, 89-100.

International Association for the Study of Pain. (1994). *Classification of chronic pain* (2nd ed.). Seattle, WA: IASP.

Jaywant, S.S., & Pai, A.V. (2003-04). A comparative study of pain measurement scales in acute burn patients. *The Indian Journal of Occupational Therapy, 35*(3), 13-17.

Kamoun, A., Yahia, A., Ksentini, H., Ghroubi, S., & Elleuch, M.H. (2017). Effect of nocturnal ingestion of melatonin on the static and dynamic balance in the elderly. *Annals of Physical and Rehabilitation Medicine, 60*, e52-e53.

Katz-Leurer, M., Fisher, I., Neeb, M., Schwartz, I., & Carmeli, E. (2009). Reliability and validity of the modified functional reach test at the sub-acute stage post-stroke. *Disability and Rehabilitation, 31*(3), 243-248.

Kirby, R.L., Swuste, J., Dupuis, D.J., MacLeod, D.A., & Monroe, R. (2002). The wheelchair skills test: A pilot study of a new outcome measure. *Archives of Physical Medicine & Rehabilitation, 83*(1), 10-18.

Kloseck, M., & Crilly, R.G. (1997). *Leisure competence measure: Professional manual and users' guide.* London, ON: Leisure Competence Measure Data System.

Kloseck, M., Crilly, R.G., & Hutchinson-Troyer, L. (2001). Measuring therapeutic recreation outcomes in rehabilitation: Further testing of the leisure competence measure. *Therapeutic Recreation Journal, 35*(1), 31-42.

Kratz, A.L., Chadd, E., Jensen, M.P., Kehn, M., & Kroll, T. (2015). An examination of the psychometric properties of the community integration questionnaire (CIQ) in spinal cord injury. *The Journal of Spinal Cord Medicine, 38*(4), 446-455.

Lynch, S.M., Leahy, P., & Barker, S.P. (1998). Reliability of measurements obtained with a modified functional reach test in subjects with spinal cord injury. *Physical Therapy, 78*(2), 130-133.

Macht, J.W., Abel, M.G., Mullineaux, D.R., & Yates, J.W. (2016). Development of 1RM prediction equations for bench press in moderately trained men. *Journal of Strength & Conditioning Research, 30*(10), 2901-2906.

Mann, D.L., Runswick, O.R., & Allen, P.M. (2016). Hand and eye dominance in sport: Are cricket batters taught to bat back-to-front? *Sports Medicine, 46*(9), 1355-1363.

Mathiowetz, V., Weber, K., Volland, G., & Kashman, N. (1984). Reliability and validity of grip and pinch strength evaluations. *Journal of Hand Surgery, 9A*, 222-226.

Miles, W.R. (1930). Ocular dominance in human adults. *Journal of General Psychology, 3*, 412-430.

Nalebuff, E., & Philips, C.A. (1990). The rheumatoid thumb. In J. Hunter, J. Schneider, E. Mackin, & A. Calla-han (Eds.), *Rehabilitation of the hand: Surgery and therapy* (3rd ed., pp. 929-941). St. Louis, MO: Mosby.

do Nascimento, M.A., Cyrino, E.S., Nakamura, F.Y., Romanzini, M., Pianca, H.J.C., & Queiroga, M.R. (2007). Validation of the Brzycki equation for the estimation of 1-RM in the bench press. *Brazilian Journal of Sporting Medicine, 13*(1), 40e-42e.

National Center on Health, Physical Activity, & Disability (NCHPAD). (2017). Fitness assessments for individuals who use a wheelchair. Toolkit for the fitness professional. Retrieved October 12, 2017, from www.nchpad.org

Newton, R.A. (2001). Validity of the multi-directional reach test: A practical measure of stability in older adults. *Journal of Gerontology: Medical Sciences, 56A*(4), M248-252.

Niewiadomski, W., Laskowska, D., Gasiorowska, A., Cybulski, G., Strasz, A., & Langfor, J. (2008). Determination and prediction of one repetition maximum (1RM): Safety considerations. *Journal of Human Kinetics, 19*, 109-120.

Pescatello, L.S., & American College of Sports Medicine. (2014). *ACSM's guidelines for exercise testing and prescription.* Philadelphia: Wolters Kluwer/Lippincott Williams & Wilkins Health.

Petersen, P., Petrick, M., Connor, H., & Conklin, D. (1989). Grip strength and hand dominance: Challenging the 10% rule. *American Journal of Occupational Therapy, 43*, 444-447.

Plummer, P., Morris, M.E., & Dunai, J. (2003). Assessment of unilateral neglect. *Physical Therapy, 83*(8), 732-740.

Podsiadlo, D., & Richardson, S. (1991). The timed up and go: A test of basic functional mobility for frail elderly persons. *Journal of the American Geriatric Society, 39*(2), 142-148.

Pollock, M.L., Miller, H.S., Linnerud, A.C., Laughridge, E., Coleman, E., & Alexander, E. (1974). Arm pedaling as an endurance training regimen for the disabled. *Archives of Physical Medicine Rehabilitation, 55*(9), 418-424.

Powell, L.E., & Myers, A.M. (1995). The activities-specific balance confidence (ABC) scale. *The Journal of Gerontology Series A: Biological Sciences and Medical Sciences, 50A*(1), M28-M34.

Rikli, R.E., & Jones, C.J. (1998). The reliability and validity of a 6-minute walk test as a measure of physical endurance in older adults. *Journal of Aging and Physical Activity, 6*, 363-375.

Rikli, R.E., & Jones, C.J. (2001). *Senior fitness test manual.* Champaign, IL: Human Kinetics.

Rikli, R.E., & Jones, C.J. (2013). Development and validation of criterion-referenced clinically relevant fitness standards for maintaining physical independence in later years. *The Gerontologist, 53*(4), 255-267.

Sawka, M.N., Foley, M.E., Pimental, N.A., Toner, M.M., & Pandolf, K.B. (1982). Arm crank protocols for determination of maximal aerobic power. *Medicine & Science in Sports & Exercise, 14*, 168.

Sisto, S.A., & Dyson-Hudson, T. (2007). Dynamometry testing in spinal cord injury. *Journal of Rehabilitation Research & Development, 44*(1), 123-136.

Skalko, T.K., Sauter, W., Burgess, L., & Loy, D.P. (2013). Assessing balance and fall efficacy in community-dwelling adults. *Therapeutic Recreation Journal, 47*(4), 291-306.

Sol, M.E., Verschuren, O., de Groot, L., de Groot, J.F., & Fit For the Future! Consortium. (2017). Development of a wheelchair mobility skills test for children and adolescents: Combining evidence with clinical expertise. *BMC Pediatrics, 17*(51), 1-18.

Stumbo, N.J. (2003). *Client assessment in therapeutic recreation services*. Urbana, IL: Sagamore.

Stumbo, N.J., & Peterson, C.A. (2009). *Therapeutic recreation program design: Principles and procedures* (5th ed.). San Francisco: Pearson.

Torhaug, T., Brurok, B., Hoff, J., Helgerudand, J., & Leivseth, G. (2016). The effect from maximal bench press strength training on work economy during wheelchair propulsion in men with spinal cord injury. *Spinal Cord, 54*, 838-842.

Turk, D.C., & Melzack, R. (Eds.). (2001). *Handbook of pain assessment* (2nd ed.). New York: The Guilford Press.

United States Census Bureau. (2010). Retrieved October 5, 2017, from www.census.gov/en.html

Ventry, I.M., & Weinstein, B.E. (1983). Identification of elderly people with hearing problems. *ASHA, 25*, 37-42.

Wells, K.F., & Dillon, E.K. (1952). The sit and reach: A test of back and leg flexibility. *Research Quarterly—American Association for Health, Physical Education and Recreation, 23*(1), 115-118.

Whiteneck, G.G., Charlifue, S.W., Frankel, H.L., Fraser, M.H., Gardner, B.P., Gerhart, K.A., et al. (1992). Mortality, morbidity, and psychosocial outcomes of persons with spinal cord injured more than 20 years ago. *Paraplegia, 20*, 617-630.

Willer, B., Ottenbacher, K.J., & Coad, M.L. (1994). The Community Integration Questionnaire: A comparative examination. *American Journal of Physical Medicine and Rehabilitation, 73*, 103-111.

Wong-Baker FACES Foundation. (2016). *Wong-Baker FACES® pain rating scale*. Retrieved October 20, 2017, from www.WongBakerFACES.org

Wong, D., & Baker, C. (1988). Pain in children: Comparison of assessment scales. *Pediatric Nursing, 14*(1), 9-17.

World Health Organization. (2001). *ICF: International classification of functioning, disability and health*. Geneva: Author.

World Health Organization. (2017). International classification of functioning, disability, and health (ICF). Retrieved September 23, 2017, from https://www.who.int/classifications/icf/en/

ADDITIONAL RESOURCES

Centers for Disease Control. (CDC, 2017). *Important facts about falls*. Retrieved October 12, 2017, from www.cdc.gov/homeandrecreationalsafety/falls/adultfalls.html

Lewald, J. (2002). Vertical sound localization in blind humans. *Neuropsychologia, 40*, 1868-1872.

Mathiowetz, V., Kashman, N., Volland, G., Weber, K., Dowe, M., & Rogers, S. (1985). Grip and pinch strength: Normative data for adults. *Archives of Physical Medicine & Rehabilitation, 66*, 69-72.

Mpofu, E., & Oakland, T. (Eds.). (2010). *Rehabilitation and health assessment: Applying ICF guidelines*. New York: Springer.

National Center on Health, Physical Activity, & Disability (NCHPAD). (2017). Fitness assessments for individuals who use a wheelchair. Toolkit for the fitness professional. Retrieved from www.nchpad.org/fitnesstesting

Rehab Institute of Chicago-Center for Rehabilitation Outcomes Research. (2017). The rehabilitation measures database. Retrieved from www.rehabmeasures.org

CHAPTER 8

Recreational Therapy Assessment and Individuals With Intellectual Disabilities

Frederick Green, PhD, CTRS

Christina Jacobs, LMSW

LEARNING OBJECTIVES

Upon completion of the text, the student will demonstrate:

- Knowledge of evidence-based recreational therapy assessment instruments used to determine physical, cognitive, emotional, and social functioning of individuals with intellectual disabilities.
- Knowledge of evidence-based assessment instruments from other health care disciplines that may be relevant to recreational therapy practice when assessing individuals with intellectual disabilities.
- Knowledge of problems and limitations that may occur with the intellectually disabled population.

The purpose of this chapter is to discuss the function of a recreational therapy assessment for effective service delivery for individuals with intellectual disabilities. The authors will first present a definition of intellectual disability with a focus on etiology and criteria for diagnosis. Next, the authors will discuss the assessment of functioning by domains as related to the WHO ICF measures of functioning, as well as the relationship of these assessments to the diagnosis of intellectual disability.

The discussion will include an understanding of assessment and adaptive behaviors, classification of intellectual disability, and evidence of problems or limitations in life activities. Participation of individuals with disabilities in life roles is presented with a special focus on inclusion, the factors that inhibit inclusion, and assessment techniques that identify strengths and supports needed to become a functioning and contributing member of one's community. Finally, environmental and personal factors that limit participation in the life of the community will be discussed.

For those of us in the therapeutic recreation profession who have been fortunate enough to have had the opportunity to work with individuals with intellectual disabilities, we recognize the multiple functions of assessment in the delivery of our services. While referring to the *International Classification of Functioning, Disability and Health* (ICF) for developing an understanding of the functioning of individuals with intellectual disabilities, we recognize that *intellectual disability* refers to a deviation from a population norm, resulting in substantial limitations in intellectual functioning and adaptive behavior (American Association on Intellectual and Developmental Disabilities, 2019). The results of the deviation may result in activity limitations, which may in turn limit one's participation in expected and desired life roles (Majnemer, 2012). Thus, assessment plays several roles. First, assessments are employed to determine if an individual has an intellectual disability and to what extent the disability exists. These assessments attempt to identify deviations from an expected norm in physiological or psychological functioning (Majnemer, 2012). A second purpose of assessment of individuals with intellectual disabilities is to help determine limitations in an individual's capacity to perform typical life tasks, or *activity skills* (Bullock & Mahon, 2017), as well as determine individual strengths that form the foundation of supports for successful life functioning (AAIDD, 2019). Pre- and post-assessment of activity task performance can provide the information necessary to identify and measure deficits in activity task skills and eventual data for determining the effectiveness of service delivery. Finally, all recreational therapists who are providing active treatment services (as well as most recreational therapy students) should recognize the importance of an assessment of the extent to which an individual is included and engaged in life activities (participation), as well as the factors that can limit participation.

Intellectual Disability Defined

In order to start the discussion on the function of recreational therapy assessments for individuals with intellectual disabilities, it may help to consider the definition of intellectual disability as a diagnostic-related group, since several related definitions of intellectual disability exist. The following characteristics are common criteria for diagnosing intellectual disability.

1. Significant impairment in cognitive functioning
2. Significant impairment in adaptive behavior
3. Occurring during the developmental period

Cognitive functioning refers to general mental capacity and includes skills such as learning, reasoning, and memory. *Adaptive behavior* is defined as a collection of functional skills used in everyday life. AAIDD also recommends that environmental factors such as community environments and culture and personal characteristics like communication skills that may affect assessment scores be considered in the assessment and diagnosis of individuals with intellectual disabilities (AAIDD, 2019).

Other definitions have been developed such as the World Health Organization (WHO, 2010), which defines intellectual disability as impaired intelligence, or a "significantly reduced ability to understand new or complex information and to learn and apply new skills" (p. 1), causing limitations that result in impaired social functioning. The definition also includes the added criteria that intellectual disability is manifested before adulthood and has a lifelong impact on an individual's development.

As noted in chapter 3, the *International Classification of Functioning, Disability and Health* offers a model to classify and understand functioning and disability from health condition through contextual factors. The following addresses the assessment of the functional domains of the individual and the integration of the ICF in relation to persons with intellectual disabilities.

Assessment and Diagnosis

When considering assessment options while working with individuals with intellectual disabilities, consider that deficits in cognitive functioning are the prime characteristic of intellectual disability. The ICF Model of Functioning and Disability can thus serve as a guideline for an assessment strategy. An assessment of body functions and structures can provide insight into the existence and potential causes of cognitive and motor limitations. Assessment in the area of activity will often look at an individual's capacity to perform life activities, including environmental and personal barriers that disrupt performance, and the strengths and resources that provide support. Assessment of an individual's capacity to participate in life activities can focus on the extent to which the individual is included and the environmental and personal factors that limit and support acceptance in the community.

Cognitive Assessment

Most likely, the initial assessment conducted with an individual with an intellectual dis-

ability is one to determine whether or not the condition of intellectual disability actually exists. Children who exhibit a developmental delay may be referred to specialists for further assessment, often for the purpose of determining whether the individual has an intellectual disability (Felix & Tymeson, 2017). The need for identifying a "label" for the condition is not without controversy. As noted by Bullock and Mahon (2017), labeling can have the negative effect of associating an individual with their disability and all of the negative preconceptions that go with it rather than focusing on the uniqueness of each individual and their inherent strengths that provide the supports for pursuing life satisfaction and engagement in the life of the community. Compounding the problem is the reliance on assessment to classify individuals based on the severity of the disability. However, assessment, identification, and labeling may serve the purpose of determining eligibility for services and could be helpful in determining the effectiveness of interventions.

The definition of and defining criteria for intellectual disability includes both deficits in cognitive abilities and limitations in functioning, as well as a criterion that the limitations are manifested before the age of 18 (Cavanaugh, 2017). Thus, the assessment of the third criterion is the most straightforward, as it would only require one to know the age of the individual when the limitations first occurred. The assessment of the other two defining criteria will often focus on what an individual does not have or what they cannot do.

The diagnostic information for identifying intellectual disability that may be of more use to the recreational therapist is reported as an IQ score, with an IQ score at least two standard deviations below the mean on a standard intelligence test like the Stanford-Binet V (Roid, 2003), the Wechsler Intelligence Scale for Children (Wechsler, 2014), or the Wechsler Adult Intelligence Scale (Wechsler, 2008) serving as the criteria line for the identification of intellectual disability (Cavanaugh, 2017). The assessment procedures for determining intellectual disability can be administered as an interview, through observations, or through formal and informal assessment procedures, and like any assessment, there are guidelines used to assure accuracy (Harrison & Oakland, 2015). The recreational therapist would not likely be the clinician administering IQ batteries. However, understanding IQ testing and results is important for professional discussions and, in this context, may be of some value in planning an intervention.

However, the definition of intelligence often varies depending on the professional who is defining it. In his quest to find a way to measure intelligence, Wechsler (1944) stated that intelligence was "the aggregate or global capacity of the individual to act purposefully, to think rationally, and to deal with their environment" (p. 3). Other characteristics of intelligence identified by experts include abstract thinking or reasoning (b164, higher-level cognitive functions), problem solving (b1646, capacity to acquire knowledge), memory (b144, memory functions including b1440, short-term memory; b1441, long-term memory; and b1442, retrieval of memory), adaptation to one's environment, mental speed, linguistic competence (b167, mental functions of language including b1670, reception of language and b1671, expression of language), mathematical competence, general knowledge, creativity, sensory acuity, goal directness (b164), and achievement motivation (Sattler, 1988; WHO, 2001). Thus, understanding these functional characteristics helps the recreational therapist better classify functioning consistent with the ICF.

Assessing Body Structure and Function

Assessment of body structure and function can focus on the cause and physical existence of factors that have produced significant limitations in intellectual functioning or may focus on the domain of physical functioning. Cavanaugh (2017) suggested that there are myriad causes of intellectual disabilities and noted that the causes are often an interaction among genetics, environment, development, trauma, and behavior. This information would allow the recreational therapist to better understand the factors that are limiting cognitive functioning and factors that could result in contraindications. For example, individuals with Down syndrome may have many possible secondary concerns of which the recreational therapist should be aware. These may include poor balance, increased risk of heart disease and respiratory problems, deficits in vision and hearing, and atlantoaxial instability, among others (Cavanaugh, 2017). This information may assist the recreational therapist in selecting the supports necessary for participation in life activities, as well as avoiding activities that may result in injury.

Assessing Motor Functioning

The assessment of motor functioning is a key element in addressing the physical domain for individuals with intellectual disability. There exist numerous assessment instruments that measure motor functioning, such as the Bruininks-Oseretsky Test of Motor Proficiency (BOT-2) (Bruininks & Bruininks, 2005; Wuang & Su, 2009).

The BOT-2 measures both fine and gross motor performance. The BOT-2 is comprised of 53 items across four motor areas: Fine Manual Control (Fine Motor Precision, seven items, and Fine Motor Integration, eight items); Manual Coordination (Manual Dexterity, five items, and Upper-Limb Coordination, seven items); Body Coordination (Bilateral Coordination, seven items, and Balance, nine items); and Strength and Agility (Running Speed and Agility, five items, and Strength, five items). Although the BOT-2 serves well to assess motor proficiency, it is not appropriate for all segments of the intellectual disability community (Bruininks & Bruininks, 2005).

In Wuang and Su's 2009 study of the validity and reliability of the BOT-2 with children with intellectual disabilities, the internal consistency of the BOT-2 total score was $a = 0.92$. This was lower than measures for children without ID in the same age range ($a = 0.95$) (Bruininks & Bruininks, 2005). However, the mean Cronbach for the subtests and composites in the Wuang and Su study were slightly higher in children with ID (0.85 and 0.88, respectively). The test-retest reliability coefficients (ICC) were excellent for the total BOT-2 and its subtests and composites with the ID subjects.

Other measures such as the Movement Assessment Battery for Children (MABC) are also used to assess motor function and movement (Brown & Lalor, 2009). It is primarily used with children with less impairment in functioning. The battery consists of four age-related item sets (ages 4 to 6, 7 to 8, 9 to 10, and 11 to 12). There are eight items for each age group. The assessment includes the following subscales: manual dexterity (three items), ball skills (two items), and static and dynamic balance (three items). A scale of 0 to 5 is used to score each item. The sum of the item scores per subscale offers a subscale score. The subscale scores can be summed for a total score for motor development ranging from 0 to 40. A high score indicates poor motor performance.

The MABC has acceptable validity and reliability for children from general classrooms and can be used for special education. Inter-rater reliability for the MABC ranges from 0.70 to 0.89 and the test-retest reliability is 0.75 (Henderson, Sugden, & Barnett, 2007). In determining the appropriateness of the MABC for diverse populations, the assessment has been used with children with Down syndrome, learning disabilities (LD), hearing impairments, and visual impairments (Brown & Lalor, 2009).

Assessment of Activity

As we develop our recreational therapy programs and design our assessment procedures to facilitate positive change, we may want to consider the focus of our efforts. An assessment that reveals a cause or a predisposition to carry the gene for intellectual disability is generally not the focus of recreational therapy assessment and services. Much of the useful information regarding body function and structure may be gleaned from the individual's individualized education plan (IEP), chart, or transition plan, negating the need for a recreational therapy assessment. The recreational therapist should therefore focus energy on areas in which they

can be effective change agents and lead the endeavor to support the efforts of individuals with intellectual disabilities to become fully functioning participants in life activities.

A functional use of assessment of individuals with intellectual disabilities may be to help determine limitations in an individual's capacity to perform typical life (or activity) tasks as well as the strengths and supports that will help them be successful (Bullock & Mahon, 2017). A good starting point will include a review of the defining criteria for intellectual disabilities, including significant deficits in adaptive behavioral skills, which are necessary for functioning in daily life activities (Cavanaugh, 2017). The assessment of adaptive behavioral skills broadly defined involves determining functioning in everyday areas, including daily living skills, social skills, independent living skills, communication, leisure, and coping skills (Lopata, Smith, Volker, Thomeer, Lee, & McDonald, 2013). Assessment of adaptive behavioral functioning is considered a critical component of comprehensive evaluations for children and adults with intellectual disabilities, because it considers the individual's functional adjustment in everyday situations (Klin, Saulnier, Tsatsanis, & Volkmar, 2005).

Activity and the ICF

Adaptive behavioral assessment scores are often reported in standard deviations from the mean. They often reflect that an individual's performance shows significant limitations and is below the expectation of a similar peer group. *Significant limitations* refer to scoring at least two standard deviations below the mean on assessments in one of three areas of adaptive behavioral skills. Adaptive behavioral skill areas include conceptual skills (d160-d179, applying knowledge, including focusing attention, thinking, reading, writing, calculating, solving problems both simple and complex, and self-direction), social skills (d710-d729, general interpersonal interactions, including d710, basic interpersonal interactions, d720, complex interpersonal interactions, and d730-d779, particular interpersonal relationships), and practical skills (d5, Self-Care) (Bullock &

Mahon, 2017; Cavanaugh, 2017; WHO, 2001). These adaptive behavioral skills represent many tasks and activities that allow individuals to perform successfully in daily life activities and respond to changes in environment (Cavanaugh, 2017).

Assessment Tools for Activity

Specific assessment tools used to evaluate adaptive behaviors vary from specific themes to overall skill areas. Two frequently used assessment tools include the Adaptive Behavior Assessment System (ABAS-III) (Harrison & Oakland, 2015) and the Vineland Adaptive Behavior Scales-Second Edition (VABS-II) (Sparrow, Cicchetti, & Balla, 2005). Both instruments assess everyday living skills for people with intellectual disabilities. The ABAS-III is designed to assess performance in daily living skills by individuals with intellectual disabilities and other conditions. Specific targeted skill domains include conceptual skills, social skills, and practical skills. Therapists, teachers, parents, and, in some cases, the individuals themselves assess the individual's capacity to function within these domains by using a four-point response scale to rate if and how frequently an individual performs these activities. This is a norm-referenced assessment. Separate assessment for activity kits are available for infants and preschoolers, school-age children, and adults.

The Vineland Adaptive Behavior Scales assesses an individual's communication, daily living skills, socialization, and motor skills. Leisure and play skills are included as a subdomain under the domain of socialization. The focus of the assessment is to determine what skills and behaviors are performed rather than focusing on capacity to perform. The assessment administrator conducts an interview with a caregiver or someone else familiar with the individual to discuss performance in current activities, and then compares these activities to those of same-age peers. Both the ABAS-III and the VABS-II require a level B qualification (a BA/BS degree in psychology, special education, or related field) by administrators. Thus, a recreational therapist will need additional and specific training to conduct these assessments.

Assessment of activity skills by a recreational therapist can serve additional functions. The classification system based on functioning in adaptive skills and the level of support needed to perform these skills are used as a method for further understanding intellectual disability (Cavanaugh, 2017). According to the 2019 AAIDD classification system, intellectual disabilities are classified according to the level of support needed to perform adaptive skills. This classification does not entirely replace the previous system of basing classification on intelligence test scores. However, identifying the supports needed to perform activities may provide more helpful information when included as part of an individual's transition plan.

Pre- and post-assessment of activity task performance (task analysis) can also provide the information necessary to identify and measure deficits in activity tasks, as well as eventual data for determining the effectiveness of service delivery. These tasks may also parallel discrete activities under the ICF. Recreational therapists who employ recreation and experiential activities as a means to an end could identify the extent of deficits in adaptive skills and use recreation and experiential-based activities to limit, minimize, or eliminate the deficits. As noted by Green, Hopper, and Singleton (2017), assessment results and evaluative data from service delivery can also be used for research purposes by generating the evidence upon which we can safely and confidently base practices with a focus on functional intervention and outcomes.

Task Analytic Assessment/ Discrepancy Analysis

A task analysis is a simple tool for assessing an individual's capacity to perform a selected behavior. It also allows the recreational therapist to identify strengths, develop a plan for instruction, and track an individual's performance over time (Schleien, Ray, & Green, 1997). A task analysis should be developed for any behavior to be learned based on expected performance. To develop a task analysis, do the following:

1. Break the behavior down into a series of steps, written as individual behavioral objectives, in the order they are to be performed.
2. Each step should consist of one behavior. The behavior in each step should be observable.
3. In some cases, a condition statement or criteria can be added.
4. Assessment is performed by prompting the individual to start the behavior and recording their performance on each step.
5. A well-written task analysis will be designed so that the successful completion of one step will serve as the natural prompt for initiating the next step.

See appendix B for an example of a task analysis.

Task/Discrepancy Analysis

A task/discrepancy analysis is similar to a task analysis. However, it includes strategies for assisting an individual with the steps or behaviors that they have difficulty with. See appendix C for an example of a task/discrepancy analysis.

Conclusions and Recommendations

As with all recreational therapy service delivery, the delivery of services for individuals with intellectual disabilities (ID) is congruent with the Comprehensive Recreational Therapy Service Delivery model (CRTSD). The assessment process and service delivery for persons with ID include the distinct actions of assessment of functional and activity skills, interests, activity analysis, task analysis, and identification of ICF codes to facilitate the ultimate goal of community engagement.

This chapter provides insights into how the assessment process for persons with ID fits well into the ICF classification system and provides a systematic process to empower a person with an intellectual disability to engage in the life of the community. Recreational therapy services must take into consideration health condition, body function and structure, and environmental and personal contextual factors in service delivery. In addition, an analysis of activity components and participation are all included in the assessment process and can be classified via the ICF. The case study at the end of the chapter provides an example that can be translated to RT practice.

Assessment and Participation

Recreational therapists who are providing recreational therapy services (as well as most recreational therapy students) recognize the importance of assessing the extent to which an individual is functioning well with life tasks (activities). An equally important assessment task is to determine the extent to which each individual is included in preferred environments as indicated by meaningful involvement in life situations (participation). While change, growth, functional improvement, and other health-related outcomes are often the focus and purpose of recreational therapy interventions, the discharge or transition goals for many individuals with intellectual disabilities are often centered on a desire to be accepted and included into personally preferred community environments and events. Community inclusion can thus be defined by the extent to which an individual participates in life situations.

In order to discuss the assessment of participation in life situations by individuals with intellectual disabilities, a comparison between *activity* and *participation* as they relate to the ICF is warranted. Peterson, Mpofu, & Oakland (2010) distinguished between "activities" functions and "participation" functions by noting that *activities* refer to carrying out tasks or actions, whereas *participation* refers to becoming involved in life situations. Bullock and Mahon (2017) refer to *participation* as engagement in life activities. Engagement, thus, can be viewed as a social construct that may be as individually defined as recreation or leisure. For example, while researching the extent to which high school students with disabling conditions were included in extramural athletic activities, Shaw and Stoll (2017) distinguished between student involvement as a player and students' perceived involvement in some other capacity, such as team manager. The authors determined that participation was often defined by programmers as participation in roles as managers rather than as active players in the sports or activities. However, in an earlier study, Eriksson and Granlund (2004) discovered that students with disabilities and parents and teachers vary in how they define participation. Students viewed participation as being part of something and a feeling of involvement, including membership on a team as a manager, whereas parents and teachers focused on the activity itself. Thus, as social constructs, inclusion and involvement in life situations may need to be individually defined.

From the perspective of a recreational therapist, and in consideration of recreation activity engagement, we might make the argument that the activities function could be assessed by measuring the extent to which an individual can perform recreation and recreation-related tasks. Assessment by recreational therapists of the participation function would measure the extent that one's activity participation is supportive of one's preferred lifestyle, which in turn supports the individual's involvement in the world around them. Thus, in this chapter, *participation* refers to inclusion through activity engagement. The concept of recreation inclusion has evolved over the years. At one time, inclusion (or the earlier terms *integration* and *mainstreaming*) was influenced by the principle of normalization (Schleien, Ray, & Green, 1997). The extent to which one was included was defined in part by the type of environment in which an individual participated, the number of nondisabled peers sharing the environment, the frequency of interactions with nondisabled peers, and the extent to which they were accepted and befriended by nondisabled peers. These are all essential and measurable goals, allowing practitioners to determine and measure inclusion and note change. However, these goals are partially based on a predetermined assumption that inclusion is a social construct that can be universally defined based on an expected norm, and thus goals for inclusion are universal.

The emergence of social role valorization as a guiding principle and a focus on person-centered planning changed the perception of inclusion from a static yet measurable norm to the recognition that inclusion, like leisure, may be a social construct that is individually defined. In a brief article in a newsletter published by the Mississippi Council on Developmental Disabilities, Green (2002) presented a five-level model of inclusion. In this model, recreation inclusion is intertwined with leisure. Accordingly, it is not the activity or the environment that determines whether someone is included, nor is it the type of people with whom one is sharing the activity. Rather, to be included means that one is participating in individually preferred life activities in personally preferred environments, and with individually preferred companions.

The author inferred that inclusion was a continuous growth process, and suggested that all individuals were working toward inclusion as defined by participation in leisure at a level that met their own needs. Additionally, inclusion, like leisure, was individually defined based on personal experience and preference. Many of the constructs that once defined inclusion (such as the percentage of individuals with disabilities participating in a group or friendships with nondisabled peers) were viewed as personal preferences and not norms. The role of the recreational therapist in the inclusion process for individuals with intellectual disabilities is to assist the individual in developing their functional and leisure skills, then using those skills to become included (as individually perceived by the individual), thus facilitating participation in life activities. The task of the recreational therapist is to assess the individual's functional capacity, the extent to which an individual is included, the extent to which they would like to be included, and the leisure and leisure-related variables that will assist them to achieve their highest level of inclusion. There are five levels of inclusion, presented as a continuum for recreational services for individuals with intellectual disabilities.

Level 1: Participating in age-appropriate, personally satisfying leisure activities.

Level 2: Making personal decisions regarding leisure.

Level 3: Participating in community recreation.

Level 4: Participating as a member of a community group.

Level 5: Becoming a contributing member of one's community.

Level 1: Participating in Age-Appropriate, Personally Satisfying Leisure Activities

The elementary level of inclusion is satisfied if an individual is either participating in at least one personally satisfying leisure activity, or receiving the necessary support to develop the skills to participate. The role of the recreational therapist is to assist an individual in selecting at least one preferred and potentially personally satisfying leisure activity and to teach the skills necessary to participate in the activity. At this level, the environment would not define the extent of inclusion, because a recreational therapist working with an individual with an intellectual disability with significant limitations and limited leisure involvement would be working toward inclusion regardless of the environment. The assessment tasks of the recreational therapist would include

1. determining the most appropriate activities to target for instruction,

2. determining interest, and

3. assessing the functional and leisure-related skills associated with participation in the activity.

Interest and preference assessments are helpful for determining interests but comprise only part of the assessment, because selected activities should be readily available to the individual (see Environmental Analysis). Con-sidering that some individuals may learn only a small number of preferred leisure activities across their lifetime, the interest and preference assessment process would need to be thorough. Once selected, recreational therapists may wish to conduct a skills assessment using the task/discrepancy analysis (see appendix C).

Level 2: Making Personal Decisions Regarding Leisure

For individuals with intellectual disabilities, progression toward inclusion through recreational activities continues as the individual begins to make personal decisions regarding leisure. Choice and preference are important defining characteristics of both leisure and inclusion. As individuals work toward inclusion, they begin to make decisions about leisure participation, including deciding in which activities to participate, when they would like to participate in the activity, and for how long. Additionally, they have choices to make, including where they would like to go for participation and with whom they would like to participate (e320, e325). Again, the environment and companions do not define the extent of inclusion; rather, the individual is building the capacity to engage in life situations by choosing activities, environments, and companions. The role of the recreational therapist is to teach adaptive and collateral skills, including decision making and consequences, time management, social skills, and how to find the resources necessary to participate in preferred leisure across multiple environments. Assessments would help identify preferred activities, potential partners, functional environments, extent of self-awareness (including strengths and limitations), and locus of control. Recreational therapists may refer to Rotter (1966) for information on assessing locus of control and may find the Rotter's Locus of Control Scale a useful instrument for assessment. A 29-item scale with scoring procedures useful for persons performing at a higher functioning level can be found online (www.mccc.edu/~jenningh/Courses/documents/Rotter-locusofcontrolhandout.pdf).

Level 3: Participating in Community Recreation

Individuals with intellectual disabilities who are progressing toward inclusion begin to apply their leisure interests and skills to identify and participate in community recreation activities of their choice. In this case, *community* is also a construct defined by the individual—it can be as small as a home or school, or as large as the individual can conceive. Inclusion is again not defined by the abilities of fellow participants but rather by the extent the individual perceives to be accepted in the environment of their choosing. For example, the individual may choose to participate in a mixed-ability art class that meets the classic definition of inclusion (d9203) or in a program entirely for individuals with disabling conditions. The fact that the program is in the community and chosen by the individual allows the individual to be working toward inclusion by accessing increasingly less restrictive environments. This level supports inclusion only if the activity and environment are truly personally chosen and not option-restricted. Assessment procedures necessary for success might include an environmental analysis for identifying potential community recreation activities, task analytic assessments and discrepancy analysis for identifying required skills and skill deficits, an interest assessment, and a social relationship assessment for identifying potential leisure partners (Schleien, Ray, & Green, 1997).

Level 4: Participating as a Member of a Community Group

It is level four where the constructs of leisure and inclusion come together and begin to fully define participation in life situations. Leisure is a state of mind, defined by each individual (Hurd & Anderson, 2011). Inclusion, likewise, becomes a state of mind, and when combined with leisure, allows an individual to develop a leisure-based identity that connects them to other like-minded people. For example, at this level, an individual begins to lose the label of an individual with an intellectual disability who plays tennis and begins to be identified as a tennis player. Tennis players have a distinct clothing style, common language, and an expected code of behavior. Their interest in the activity of tennis, along with their tennis-related skills, will draw them together with other tennis players, as the identifying focus on disability gives way to a shared focus on tennis. Roles in this shared community are individually determined and can include playing, managing, and supporting as determined by each individual. The specific role is not as important as a perceived sense of belonging. This identity and the resultant social connections centered on shared leisure experiences serve as a conduit to participation in life situations. The role of the recreational therapist is to assist the individual to construct an identity based on interests (rather than on disabling condition) and to build the capacity to develop the adaptive skills, leisure interests, and leisure-related skills that will facilitate a sense of belonging. Assessments will focus not only on personal contextual factors that inhibit successful participation but also on environmental factors as well (see ICF and Environmental Factors). Recreational therapists would need to assess the tennis "environment," gathering the information necessary to understand not only the skills necessary to play but also the social and behavioral expectations that are necessary for becoming accepted.

Level 5: Becoming a Contributing Member of One's Community

An often overlooked aspect of the discussion on the inclusion of individuals with intellectual disabilities is the untapped potential for giving back. In this leisure-based model of inclusion, "giving back" would come in the form of using one's leisure interests and sense of identity to become a contributing member of the community. Giving back is an extension of the leisure-strengthened identity. The tennis player noted previously would have many potential opportunities to use their leisure-based activities and interests to give back. Perceiving one-self to be a tennis player opens opportunities for teaching tennis lessons, providing support at tournaments, assisting with the maintenance of courts, and the like. These tasks can result in a strengthened environmental perception of value and a personal sense of belonging. The task of the recreational therapist again focuses not only on personal factors, such as strengthening interpersonal skills and assertiveness, but also on environmental factors. Attitude assessments, followed by appropriate preparation and training of group members, may help facilitate the inclusion process.

Assessment and the Environment

According to Majnemer (2012), assessment of individuals with intellectual disabilities will often measure and subsequently distinguish between an individual's *capacity* to perform certain activity tasks and participate in life roles and their actual *ability* to perform and participate. The difference between capacity and performance is often influenced by contextual factors that interact with the individual and limit functioning (Peterson, Mpofu, & Oakland, 2010). In the ICF, these environmental factors are perceived as either a barrier or a facilitator for engagement (WHO, 2001). Bullock and Mahon (2017) noted that *disablement* (aka the impairment, activity, and participant restrictions that limit functioning) was the result of a combination of internal and external factors. These contextual factors are referred to as *environmental and personal factors* within the ICF.

ICF and Environmental Factors

Environmental factors that restrict (barrier) or promote (facilitator) activity performance and participation refer to areas such as Products and Technology (e1), Natural Environment and Human-Made Changes to Environment (e2), Support and Relationships (e3), Attitudes (e4), and Services, Systems and Policies (e5) (WHO, 2001). These environments have the potential to support an individual's effort to perform, and thus feel included, or restrict and create barriers to functioning, access, and engagement. Environmental factors would include environments in which the individual lives, works, plays, learns, and socializes, and the people with whom they interact. One role of the recreational therapist is to assess the environments in order to identify factors that may inhibit participation, as well as factors that enable and support functioning at one's preferred level of inclusion.

A growing number of assessment instruments can be used to assess the physical environment. Bullock and Mahon (2017) offer an accessibility survey in their text on community recreation services for individuals with disabilities. The survey is a checklist that allows reviewers to assess physical environments for accessibility, identify problem areas, and offer potential solutions. An environmental analysis (Schleien, Ray, & Green, 1997) is a useful assessment tool for identifying potential leisure and recreation opportunities. For the environmental analysis, the recreational therapist surveys an individual's physical environment, beginning with areas in and close to home and eventually expanding out to the community, to identify potential leisure and recreation activities and opportunities. The result of the environmental analysis is an interest assessment instrument that is personalized for one's environment. A sample interest assessment developed as a result of an environmental analysis is provided in appendix D.

Social environmental factors that may influence participation in activities and life roles include networks of friends and acquaintances, peer and family support, quality of relationships, attitudes of the public, and outside service agencies. However, assessing social environmental factors can be a little complicated. As noted by Lippold and Burns (2009), the quality of social networks (e325, acquaintances, peers, colleagues, neighbours and community members) are often assessed by looking at both the number of individuals identified in a network, as well as the characteristics of the members. In their research, the authors distinguished between the structure of the social networks, such as size and density of the network, and the function or purpose of the relationships. They noted that not only did adults with intellectual disabilities have smaller social networks with fewer friends than their peers without disabilities, but their network of perceived friends was comprised largely of care providers.

This finding was similar to the findings of Green, Schleien, MacTavish, and Benepe (1995), who concluded that the nature of social relationships constructed by individuals with intellectual disabilities may be different than social relationship patterns as perceived by their nondisabled peers. Yet they observed that social networks, if personally perceived as positive or supportive, can provide the social support necessary for meaningful participation. In their study, the authors utilized the Social Relations Assessment Procedure (Schleien, Green, & Heyne, 1993; Schleien, Ray, Green, & Heyne, 1997), which is designed to generate information that can be used to identify social relationships across nine categories (table 8.1). Specifically, the procedure is designed to assess the existence, functions, and purposes of social relationships (Schleien, Green, & Heyne, 1993). For the assessment, the recreational therapist assists the individual in identifying all of the individuals who play a role in their life. The recreational therapist then classifies each identified respondent as a *friend*, *acquaintance*, or *service provider* based on the role they play in the individual's life. Continued and in-depth discussion allows the recreational therapist to further classify the identified names in each category according to the frequency, quality, and function of the relationship. The Social Relationship Assessment Procedure is intended to allow the recreational therapist to track changes in the social relationships of each individual, as well as assist the individual in identifying potential partners for leisure participation.

The identified individuals are then "mapped" according to the function and quality of the relationships (Schleien, Ray, Green, & Heyne, 1997).

Finally, a Sociometry Evaluation Tool allows the recreational therapist to identify members of an enclosed social environment who would best provide the necessary social support for successful inclusion (Schleien, Ray, Green, & Heyne, 1997). In this procedure, the recreational therapist asks each member of the group to identify individuals that they would choose to include or exclude from their social groups. The individuals with intellectual disabilities can then be placed in groups with other individuals that offer support.

The extent to which an individual with an intellectual disability functions well in life activities and participates in life roles is also influenced by personal contextual factors. Peterson, Mpofu, and Oakland (2010) noted that personal contextual factors include personal characteristics such as "gender, race, age, fitness, religion, lifestyle, upbringing, coping styles, experiences, behavior patterns, psychological assets, etc." (p. 14). These contextual characteristics are also included in the ICF (WHO, 2001). Many of these characteristics are partially included within diversity domains that identify minority status (Allison & Schneider, 2008), whereas membership in any minority group may influence an individual's ability to participate in life activities. For individuals with intellectual disabilities, the personal characteristics that result from the impairment will also have an impact on participation. The challenge with these personal characteristics is that they are difficult to classify and are individually defined (WHO, 2001).

According to Cavanaugh (2017), a defining characteristic of intellectual disability is limitations in cognitive functioning. As a result, indi-

TABLE 8.1   Social Relationships

Friends	Acquaintances	Service providers
Significant other	Frequent acquaintances	Big Brothers Big Sisters
Best friends	Acquaintances	Service providers
Friends	Distant acquaintances	Care providers

viduals with intellectual disabilities may have deficits related to learning. The limitations in learning may then reduce the ability to develop the skills needed to perform related adapted behaviors and activities, and eventually limit the ability to participate in life roles. There are, however, several ramifications associated with limitations in cognitive functioning. Although people with intellectual disabilities are capable of learning, learning may occur at a slower rate (Cavanaugh, 2017). As a result, individuals may fall behind their peers and learn fewer leisure activity skills. Recreational therapists who are working with individuals on inclusion should recognize that shared leisure activities and related skills and behaviors are learned, and participants with and without intellectual disabilities can thus benefit from instruction. Those participants with intellectual disabilities may simply need more instruction and more time for learning. It may help the inclusion process to spend more time teaching skills that would enhance inclusion. Additionally, individuals with intellectual disabilities may face difficulty with learning as a result of reduced attention span (Cavanaugh, 2017). It is important to be cognizant of the individual's attention span and the resultant ability to attend to tasks, so modifications may be required, such as shorter instructional periods and more opportunities for developing skills through guided repetition (b140-b189, specific mental functions).

Cognition and Social Functioning and the ICF

Finally, individuals with intellectual disabilities may have difficulty with understanding abstract concepts (b164) (Cavanaugh, 2017; WHO, 2001). The ability to think abstractly allows one to process knowledge and experiences and create responses to varying environmental cues. Limitations in abstract thinking may make it difficult to generalize learned skills to new environments (d160-d179, applying knowledge). Perhaps more significantly, limited abstract thinking skills may make it more difficult to fit in and be included socially, because social skills and resultant behaviors

are fairly complex. Cues that are intended to elicit a social response often vary according to the social setting and situation and are not always presented in an overt, clearly defined manner (d7, Interpersonal Interactions and Relationships). Recipients of social cues may have to consider many changing variables as they prepare to respond.

For the recreational therapist, assessment of the person with an intellectual disability should consider the personal contextual factors that may limit the performance of activities and eventual participation in life roles, as well as the individual's strengths and abilities that may enhance their performance. Interventions should focus on assisting individuals to build the capacity to participate in life roles. Consider the following:

1. When assisting in the process of selecting activities, recognize the right of the individual to have ownership of the selection process. Decisions that affect an individual should be made with the individual and not for the individual.

2. Individuals who learn at a greatly reduced rate (d130-159, basic learning) may only fully learn a few leisure skills across a lifetime. Thus, the process for determining preferred activities to be targeted for instruction is critical. This process may take time.

3. While assessing for individual preference (d177, making decisions), recognize that reductions in abstract thinking skills (b164, higher-level cognitive functions) may make it more difficult to make complicated choices. Additionally, traditional methods of assessment may be ineffective; presenting a verbal description of an activity may not be as effective as participating in an activity for determining preference. For example, providing two or three activities or toys in a distraction-free environment and observing the individual's response can offer the therapist insights into preferred options.

4. In preparation for instruction, a task/discrepancy analysis (see appendix C) allows the recreational therapist to break

down complex tasks into observable, and eventually teachable, concrete tasks (b1641, organization and planning) (Schleien, Ray, & Green, 1997). A thorough assessment will also allow the therapist to determine abilities as well as limitations in order to classify functioning utilizing the ICF. The analysis will allow the therapist to establish learning outcomes, apply interventions, and track progress.

CASE STUDY
Laura's Transition From High School to Community Living

Instructions: The following case study is provided as a means to gain a better understanding of the use of the ICF in classifying functioning. As you read the case study, look up the functional classification codes and the associated performance codes from the ICF. Some items require that you note the functional area and look up the corresponding code.

Laura is a 20-year-old female student with an intellectual disability attending the local public high school. She lives at home with her mother and her three siblings—two sisters (one older, one younger) and her younger brother (e310+4). Laura's intellectual disability is believed to be the result of a lack of oxygen to the brain during fetal development (b117.1). Prior to starting high school, Laura's IQ was determined to be 58, or nearly three standard deviations below the mean on the Wechsler Test for Intelligence. This score would place Laura in the area of mild intellectual disability on the older AAMR classification system.

Follow-up assessments revealed that Laura had age-related deficits in adaptive behaviors. She had limited leisure interests and limited ability to share her interests with others, assessed mild limitations in self-direction (d570.1) and personal decision making (d177.1), deficits in social skills (specifically difficulty with asserting herself and making decisions) (b1266.3, d177.2), and an assessed limited network of friends and social supports (e320.2, e325.2). Most of her deficits are mild to moderate, and, in most functional areas, Laura can benefit from an intermittent level of support, because she often can learn the skills necessary to participate in many life functions (d230.2). As a result of her assessments, Laura was diagnosed with an intellectual disability, and it was determined that she was eligible for special education services because she met the following IDEA defining characteristics:

1. Significantly subaverage intellectual functioning
2. Assessed deficits in ability to perform everyday life activities (adaptive behavior) (d230, carrying out daily routine)
3. Limitations that are manifested in the developmental period (prior to the age of 18)
4. Limitations that negatively affect her school performance (d820, school education)

As a student who meets the criteria for placement in special education services, Laura is eligible for an individualized education plan (IEP) that supports her (and her family's) desire for an education in the least restrictive environment, and one that is deemed appropriate for her needs. Because of her age, Laura is attending school on campus at the local university rather than in the high school. Although her classes are primarily in a room that is separate from the university classrooms utilized for college courses, Laura has regular access to the university dining hall, library, recreation facility, and student social events.

Because this is Laura's last year of high school, her IEP focuses on plans to prepare her for making the transition from high school to adult life in the community. Her teachers are especially focusing on preparing Laura to find and hold a job in the community (d8450.2, seeking employment) and developing the daily living skills necessary for independent living (d230.2, carrying out daily routines). She is currently working on many job-related skills, including improving her interpersonal communication skills (d720.2), developing a sense of personal responsibility (d2400.2), and learning specific work tasks (d8451.1). As part of her educational program, Laura works regularly at a part-time paid student work position on campus checking student IDs at the dining hall. The plan is for Laura to apply for a job near her house and begin the process of learning the work tasks prior to graduation as part of her transition plan.

At her IEP meeting at the beginning of her last year with the high school, Laura's mom and her teacher talked with Laura about adding a leisure plan to help prepare her for her transition from school to adult life in the community. Laura's teacher felt that her work training was progressing well, and she was developing the skills and support that would aid her in maintaining her own residence. However, she realized that without a plan for leisure, Laura may be unprepared for participating in leisure activities in the community during her nonwork time (d910.3). This void may lead to Laura becoming overly sedentary (d230.3), and also may result in her becoming disconnected socially from her friends and the community (e325.2).

Laura, her mom, and her teacher met with Ed, the recreational therapist from the city's park and recreation program. Several years ago, Ed had reached out to the schools in an effort to provide recreational therapy services to students and had developed a program that supported inclusion. He explained that developing a leisure plan for transition was as involved as developing a plan for employment, and equally as important. As he explained to Laura, employment is important not only for providing the financial resources needed for living independently but also for creating and maintaining a personal identity and a sense of self-esteem. However, developing a good and satisfying lifestyle that included leisure participation would allow Laura to develop a personal identity based on leisure interests, thus helping her connect with friends and develop a sense of belonging in the community. These connections would allow her to participate in the community at increasingly higher levels and contribute to improved health and self-esteem. He explained that there were many benefits to developing a healthy lifestyle that included a range of activities, and she, along with her mom, her teacher, and the school's recreational therapist, could work collaboratively to determine the benefits most appropriate for her. Finally, he explained that a healthy lifestyle that included leisure activities was important during a time of transition. In school, Laura had developed her identity as a student, and this persona helped keep her socially active and connected with friends and peers. Once she leaves school, this identity and the social connections associated with it may be lost. By pursuing personally desired leisure activities, and identifying and overcoming the personal and environmental contextual factors that may inhibit her efforts, Laura could develop a personal leisure identity that would enable her to connect to networks of like-minded peers.

As Ed began to work with Laura, he initiated a series of assessments to help identify her restrictions to participation in activities and life events, as well as the direction she would like her leisure plan to take. The series of assessments began with the World Health Organization Disability Assessment Schedule 2.0 (WHODAS 2.0). The WHODAS 2.0 assesses functional ability associated with mental disorders and generates a global disability score as well as six domain scores, including scores in the domains of getting along with others, participation in society, and participation in life activities (Konecky, Meyer, Marx, Kimbrel, & Morisette, 2014). These domain scores are used to identify deficits as well as track changes. Ed continued with a series of assessments that are designed to produce information he found necessary to guide her program. These assessments include the following.

A Leisure Needs Assessment

For Laura's leisure needs assessment, Ed discussed with Laura what she envisioned as preferred leisure outcomes. Ed's assessment identified appropriate outcomes, presented in clusters according to the domains of health (physical, cognitive, emotional, social, or leisure). For example, Laura could choose to lose weight (physical domain) (b530), meet new people

> continued

(social domain) (d9205), or develop new leisure skills (leisure domain) (d920). Additionally, the assessment included some open-ended questions about Laura's past and current leisure interests, people with whom she would like to share time, and Laura's perception of her strengths and concerns related to leisure. The assessment instrument shown in figure 8.1 is an in-house assessment that is used in leisure education and school-based therapeutic recreation programs. It has not been published but has been presented at several conferences, including CTRA's 2018 conference.

Individual Needs

What would you like to see your son/daughter get from an individualized recreation program?

Leisure

___ New skill
___ Improve skill
___ Lifestyle change
___ Personal growth
___ Try new experiences
___ Have fun
___ Connect with community
___ Contribute to community
___ Other

Cognitive

___ Short-term memory
___ Long-term memory
___ Decision making
___ Attention
___ Reading/Writing
___ Adding/Subtracting
___ Communication
___ Problem solving
___ Other

Social

___ Meet people
___ Make friend(s)
___ Interact with new people
___ Interact with friend(s)
___ Improve social skills
___ Assertiveness
___ Other

Affective

___ Self-esteem
___ Self-efficacy
___ + Mood
___ – Aggressive behavior
___ Other

Physical

___ Lose weight
___ Gain weight
___ Strength
___ Endurance
___ Flexibility
___ Fine motor
___ Gross motor
___ Hand/Eye coordination
___ Other

FIGURE 8.1 Leisure needs assessment: Parent's version.

Adapted by permission from R. Green, *Including Students with Disabilities in High School Recreation and Sport Activities: Role of the Recreational Therapist in the Inclusion Process.* Paper presented at the Canadian Therapeutic Recreation Association 22nd Annual Conference (Halifax, Nova Scotia, Canada, 2018).

A Leisure Needs Follow-Up Assessment

Ed followed up his needs assessment with Laura by asking her mother and her teacher similar questions. He believed that the information he received could help him confirm the direction of Laura's preferred program. Additionally, he believed that her mother and teacher may be able to provide information that Laura had forgotten.

Environmental Analysis

In preparation for helping Laura select activities that would form the core of her leisure engagement, Ed conducted an analysis of Laura's living environment. First, Ed visited her home and identified everything in the house and on the immediate property that may be useful in her leisure plan. He found a TV with a DVD player, a saxophone, a bookshelf full of novels, an old Polaroid camera, and a box with games. He also listed some of the items in the kitchen, such as the stove, oven, and microwave, which have the potential for leisure time activities. In the garage, he found a couple of bicycles and a tennis racket. It is important to note that when identifying potential recreation options, Ed did not consider Laura's gender, age, or disability, as these considerations would come later.

Ed repeated this process as he worked his way further from Laura's house. He identified potential leisure activities within a short walking distance from her house, then a long walk or bike ride, and anything else within a three-mile radius, and then finally some major recreation facilities and activities within the small community. He especially focused on recreation clubs or groups that were actively participating in the community.

Finally, Ed assessed the available transportation options by identifying public transportation, sidewalks, bike lanes, and the general safety of neighborhoods for walking. All in all, Ed was able to identify nearly 80 potential recreation activities and groups for Laura to choose from.

Activity Analysis

Ed now had a list of 80 potential recreation activities and groups that were available to Laura. However, he realized that as a result of her disability, Laura had moderate difficulty with making decisions (d177.2), especially when there were too many options. Thus, he conducted a brief activity analysis based on Laura's earlier identified needs and preferences. For example, since Laura had moderate difficulty losing weight (b530) and desired this as a preferred outcome, he was able to identify the activities that would support this outcome. This narrowed the options a little. As he considered all of her preferences, he could cross reference and look for activities that favored many behavioral outcomes identified in the activity analysis. This procedure was not intended to eliminate options for her but to help her select activities by knowing which options would support her goals.

Interest Assessment

Ed now had a list of recreation activities and groups that were available to Laura, prioritized by the potential of each one to meet her assessed needs. These options could be presented to Laura to help her choose the ones that she would like to pursue. Several options exist for helping her make these determinations. By working closely with Laura, her mother, and her teacher, Ed was able to determine the most effective method. Ed has the option of allowing Laura to read a description of the options available to her or to have someone read the descriptions to her. He also has the option of showing her pictures or telling her more details. Finally, though, Ed finds he is able to get a better understanding of Laura's leisure interests and preferences by allowing Laura to try the activities and observing her reaction to them.

Social Relations Assessment

The Social Relations Assessment Procedure (Schleien, Green, & Heyne, 1993) is a simple, criterion-referenced assessment procedure designed to map out an individual's network of social relationships by type and function. The results of the assessment are especially useful when included as part of a transition plan because transitions can result in disruptions in relationships. The "mapping" of relationships by type and function can help the therapist on the receiving end of the transition plan prepare the individual to begin developing a new network of friends (d750).

Ed assessed Laura's network by interviewing Laura, her mom, and her teacher. He asked them to identify everyone in Laura's life with whom she has been in contact over the past three years and to describe the role they play in her life and the function of their relationship.

> continued

He then divided all responses into one of three categories: friends, acquaintances, and service providers. Ed distinguished service providers as individuals whose primary function was to provide some type of service for Laura. He distinguished between friends and acquaintances by noting that friendships include an element of mutual liking, the functions of the relationships are equally shared, and the partners in a friendship often share mutually satisfying leisure experiences. Ed then further mapped the network into three friendship categories, three acquaintance categories, and three levels of service providers.

Task/Discrepancy Analysis

The final assessment selected by Ed was a combined task/discrepancy analysis (Schleien, Ray, & Green, 1997). For each community leisure activity selected by Laura, Ed developed a thorough task analysis. He assessed Laura by prompting her to perform the steps of the task analysis and noting her ability to perform the steps and any discrepancies between the required step and her ability to perform. From this assessment, Ed could develop goals and objectives to be included in the transition plan.

Summary

To have an intellectual disability means that an individual has deficits in cognitive functioning. Assessment of body structures and functions can confirm the diagnosis, identify possible causes, and provide a classification of the disability based on the extent limitations. This information has limited value to the recreational therapist. An assessment of activity, or the capacity of the individual to complete activities necessary for daily living, may provide more functional information for the purpose of planning. The therapist may be more interested in determining the extent to which an individual is able to perform daily tasks, including participating in preferred and desired leisure activities. Additionally, a well-planned assessment will help identify the environmental and personal barriers that limit participation and the levels of support that can enhance performance.

Finally, recreational therapists should recognize the challenges an individual with intellectual disability faces when attempting to become included and trying to maximize their involvement in life situations. Assessments of personal contextual factors can help determine an individual's preferences in relationship to leisure activities, their perceived personal preference for inclusion, their strengths, and their personal limitations. Likewise, assessment of environmental factors that affect participation in life activities can identify barriers such as inaccessibility, as well as help identify potential social connections that can support efforts for inclusion. In sum, the existence of a diagnosis of intellectual disability may have an impact on life participation. However, it is the role of the recreational therapist to identify and develop the strengths and supports that may be the key to successful participation in life activities.

REFLECTION QUESTIONS

1. The classification of intellectual disability was once based on IQ scores and resulted in labels ranging from mild to profound. Now classification is often based on the support needed to perform life activities. What factors influenced this change? What are some advantages and disadvantages for recreational therapists in classifying support needed? Discuss how this change can assist with individual program development and transition services.

2. Assume that you are the recreational therapist at a community recreation facility that provides inclusion support for individuals with disabilities. The facility is a publicly funded program that is part of the community park and recreation department. You are now working with a young adult with an intellectual disability who has just moved from another state. This individual would like to become a "participating member of the community." Where do you start? What information would you need in order to begin developing a program for her? How would you obtain this information? How would you use this information to assist her with developing a sense of belonging, becoming included, and meeting her goal of participating in life events?

3. From your own experiences, identify some environmental contextual factors that may inhibit participation in life activities for a young adult with an intellectual disability. How do these factors inhibit participation in life events, and how would you measure them? What strategies can be used to minimize the barriers and enable active participation?

4. From your own experiences, identify some personal contextual factors that served as barriers to participation in life activities for a young adult with an intellectual disability. How do these factors inhibit inclusion, and how would you measure them? Why would you measure them? What strategies can be used to minimize the barriers and allow participation?

REFERENCES

Allison, M.T., & Schneider, I.E. (2008). *Diversity and the recreation profession: Organizational perspectives* (Rev. ed.). State College, PA: Venture.

American Association on Intellectual and Developmental Disabilities. (2019). Definition of intellectual disability. Retrieved from https://aaidd.org/intellectual-disability/definition

Brown, T., & Lalor, A. (2009). The Movement Assessment Battery for Children—Second Edition (MABC-2): A review and critique. *Physical & Occupational Therapy in Pediatrics, 29*(1), 86-103. doi:10.1080/01942630802574908

Bruininks, R.H., & Bruininks, B.D. (2005). *Bruininks-Oseretsky test of motor proficiency* (2nd ed.). Minneapolis, MN: Pearson Assessment.

Bullock, C.C., & Mahon, M.J. (2017). *Introduction to recreation services for people with disabilities: A person-centered approach* (4th ed.). Urbana, IL: Sagamore.

Cavanaugh, L.K. (2017). Intellectual disabilities. In J.P. Winnick & D.L. Poretta (Eds.), *Adapted physical education and sport* (6th ed., pp. 153-174). Champaign, IL: Human Kinetics.

Eriksson, L., & Granlund, M. (2004). Conceptions of participation in students with disabilities and persons in their close environment. *Journal of Developmental and Physical Disabilities, 16*, 229-245.

Felix, M., & Tymeson, G. (2017). Measurement assessment and program evaluation. In J.P. Winnick & D.L. Poretta (Eds.), *Adapted physical education and sport* (6th ed., pp. 59-78). Champaign, IL: Human Kinetics.

Green, F.P. (2002). Inclusion hierarchy. Editorial featured in *Mississippi Council on Developmental Disabilities Newsletter, 17*, p. 3.

Green, F.P., Hopper, T.D., & Singleton, J.F. (2017). Perspective: Cross collaboration in therapeutic recreation: Future implications. In N. Stumbo (Ed.), *Professional issues in therapeutic recreation* (3rd ed., pp. 579-589). Champaign, IL: Sagamore.

Green, F.P., Schleien, S.J., MacTavish, J., & Benepe, S. (1995). Nondisabled adults' perceptions of relationships in early stages of arranged partnerships with peers with mental retardation. *Education and Training in Mental Retardation and Developmental Disabilities, 30*, 91-108.

Green, R. (2018). Including students with disabilities in high school recreation and sport activities: Role of the recreational therapist in the inclusion process. Paper presented at the Canadian Therapeutic Recreation Association 22nd Annual Conference, Halifax, Nova Scotia, Canada.

Harrison, P., & Oakland, T. (2015). *Adaptive behavior assessment system (manual)* (3rd ed.). San Antonio, TX: Psychological Corporation.

Henderson, S.E., Sugden, D.A., & Barnett, A.L. (2007). *Movement assessment battery for children—second edition* [Movement ABC-2]. London, UK: The Psychological Corporation.

Hurd, A.R., & Anderson, D.M. (2011). *The park and recreation professional's handbook*. Champaign, IL: Human Kinetics. Retrieved from https://us.humankinetics.com/products/park-and-recreation-professionals-handbook-with-online-resource-the

IDEA Partnership. (2017). Part B (ages 6-21). Categories of disability under IDEA law. Retrieved from www.ideapartnership.org/topics-database/idea-2004/idea-2004-part-b/1397-definitions-of-disability-terms.html

Klin, A., Saulnier, C., Tsatsanis, K., & Volkmar, F.R. (2005). Clinical evaluation in autism spectrum disorders: Psychological assessment within a transdisciplinary framework. In F.R. Volkmar, R. Paul, A. Klin, & D. Cohen (Eds.), *Handbook of autism and pervasive developmental disorders* (pp. 772-798). Hoboken, NJ: John Wiley.

Konecky, B., Meyer, E.C., Marx, B.P., Kimbrel, N.A., & Morisette, S.B. (2014). Using the WHODAS 2.0 to assess functional disability associated with mental disorder. *American Journal of Psychiatry, 171*, 818-820. Retrieved from www.ncbi.nlm.nih.gov/pmc/articles/PMC5032648/

Lippold, T., & Burns, J. (2009). Social support and intellectual disabilities: A comparison between social networks of adults with intellectual disability and those with physical disability. *Journal of Intellectual Disability Research, 53*, 463-473.

Lopata, C., Smith, R.A., Volker, M.A., Thomeer, M.L., Lee, G.K., & McDonald, C.A. (2013). Comparison of adaptive behavior measures for children with HFASDs. *Autism Research and Treatment, 2013*, 1-10.

Majnemer, A. (2012). The purpose and framework for this text. In A. Majnemer (Ed.), *Measures for children with developmental disabilities: An ICF-CY approach* (pp. 10-15). London, UK: Mac Keith.

Peterson, D.B., Mpofu, E., & Oakland, T. (2010). Concepts and models in disability, functioning, and health. In E. Mpofu & T. Oakland (Eds.), *Rehabilitation and health assessment: Applying ICF guidelines* (pp. 3-26). New York, NY: Springer.

Roid, G.H. (2003). *Stanford-Binet intelligence scales* (5th ed.). Itasca, IL: Riverside.

Rotter, J. (1966). Generalized expectancies for internal versus external control of reinforcement. *Psychological Monographs, 80*(1), 1-12.

Sattler, J. (1988). *Assessment of children* (3rd ed.). San Diego, CA: Jerome M. Sattler.

Schleien, S.J., Green, F.P., & Heyne, L. (1993). Recreation for persons with severe handicaps. In M.E. Snell (Ed.), *Systematic instruction of persons with severe handicaps* (4th ed., pp. 526-555). Columbus, OH: Merrill.

Schleien, S.J., Ray, M.T., & Green, F.P. (1997). *Community recreation and people with disabilities: Strategies for inclusion*. Baltimore, MD: Paul H. Brookes.

Schleien, S.J., Ray, M.T., Green, F.P., & Heyne, L. (1997). Friendship. In S.J. Schleien, M.T. Ray, & F.P. Green (Eds.), *Community recreation and people with disabilities: Strategies for inclusion* (pp. 129-150). Baltimore, MD: Paul H. Brookes.

Shaw, A.H., & Stoll, S.K. (2017, August 9). Disabilities, play and possibilities [Webinar]. SHAPE America. Retrieved from http://sa.mycrowdwisdom.com/diweb/mylearning

Sparrow, S.S., Cicchetti, D.V., & Balla, D.A. (2005). *Vineland adaptive behavior scales* (2nd ed.). Circle Pines, MN: American Guidance Service.

U.S. Department of Health and Human Services. (2000). The Developmental Disabilities Assistance and Bill of Rights Act of 2000.

Vuijk, P.J., Hartman, E., Scherder, E., & Visscher, C. (2010, November). Motor performance of children with mild intellectual disability and borderline intellectual function. *Journal of Intellectual Disabilities Research, 54*, 955-965.

Wechsler, D. (1944). *The measurement of adult intelligence* (3rd ed.). Baltimore: Williams & Wilkins.

Wechsler, D. (2008). *Wechsler adult intelligence scale–fourth edition: Technical and interactive manual*. San Antonio, TX: The Psychology Corporation.

Wechsler, D. (2014). *Wechsler intelligence scale for children* (5th ed.). Bloomington, MN: Pearson.

World Health Organization. (2001). *International classification of functioning, disability and health*. Geneva, Switzerland: Author.

World Health Organization. (2010). Definition: Intellectual disability. Retrieved from www.euro.who.int/en/health-topics/noncommunicable-diseases/mental-health/news/news/2010/15/childrens-right-to-family-life/definition-intellectual-disability

Wuang, Y.P., & Su, C.Y. (2009). Reliability and responsiveness of the Bruininks-Oseretsky Test of Motor Proficiency-Second Edition in children with intellectual disability. *Research in Developmental Disabilities, 30*(5), 847-855.

ADDITIONAL RESOURCES

Council on Developmental Disabilities. (1990). The Developmental Disabilities Assistance and Bill of Rights Act: Legislative history of the act—The 1970 amendments. Retrieved from https://mn.gov/mnddc/dd_act/documents/FEDREG/90-DDA-LEGLISLATIVEHISTORY.pdf

Green, F.P. (2002). Inclusive recreation services and health-related outcomes. Paper presented at the National Institute on Recreation Inclusion Annual Conference, Las Vegas, NV, September, 2002.

Green, F.P., Schleien, S.J., MacTavish, J., & Benepe, S. (1995). Nondisabled adults' perceptions of relationships in early stages of arranged partnerships with peers with mental retardation. *Education and Training in Mental Retardation and Developmental Disabilities, 30*, 91-108.

Hoyt, J. (1987). The Senate Subcommittee on the Handicapped: Hearing on the reauthorization of the Developmental Disabilities Act of 1984. Retrieved from https://babel.hathitrust.org/cgi/pt?id=pst.000012021383;view=1up;seq=212

Nordvik, J.E., Walle, K.E., Nyberg, C.K., Fjell, A.M., Walhovd, K.B., Westlye, L.T., & Tornas, S. (2014). Bridging the gap between clinical neuroscience and cognitive rehabilitation: The role of cognitive training, models of neuroplasticity and advanced neuroimaging in future brain injury rehabilitation. *NeuroRehabilitation, 34*(1), 81-85.

Simeonsson, R.J., Sauer-Lee, A., Granlund, M., & Bjorck-Akesson, E.M. (2010). Developmental and health assessments in rehabilitation with the ICF for children and youth. In E. Mpofu & T. Oakland (Eds.), *Rehabilitation and health assessment: Applying ICF guidelines* (pp. 27-46). New York, NY: Springer.

Sprour, M., & Shevell, M.I. (2012). Genetic testing. In A. Majnemer (Ed.), *Measures for children with developmental disabilities: An ICF-CY approach* (pp. 27-36). London, UK: Mac Keith.

Volker, M.A., Lopata, C., Smerbeck, A.M., Knoll, V.A., Thomeer, M.L., Toomey, J.A., & Rodgers, J.D. (2010). BASC-2 PRS profiles for students with high-functioning autism spectrum disorders. *Journal of Autism and Developmental Disorders, 40*(2), 188-199.

CHAPTER 9

Assessing Clients With Diverse Cultural Backgrounds

Shinichi Nagata, PhD, CTRS • Tristan Hopper, PhD, CTRS

Marc Zaremski, MS, CTRS

LEARNING OBJECTIVES

Upon completion of the text, the student will demonstrate:

- Knowledge of culture and reasons why awareness of culture matters.
- Knowledge of foundational concepts that influence client behaviors.
- Knowledge of factors associated with client misunderstandings of assessment questions.
- Knowledge of the factors associated with therapist misunderstandings of client behaviors.
- Knowledge of cultural competency and cultural safety.

Have you ever traveled to a foreign country? Can you imagine getting medical treatment in that country? What if the health care providers cannot speak your language? What if they do not understand something you think is important? As you can imagine, receiving medical care in a completely foreign environment may pose challenges. In addition, it might be upsetting or disappointing if the medical service providers do not respect what you think is important. This is a common narrative of a medical service recipient who has a different cultural background.

Defining Culture

The challenges you may have imagined were all related to culture—but what is culture? Cultural sociologist Wendy Griswold (2013) defined *culture* as shared norms, values, beliefs, or expressive symbols within a group of people. The groups can be of the same nationality, ethnicity, race, and indigeneity. Some examples of culture can be food, language (e.g., British-English, Thai, Tagalog), a form of greeting (e.g., bowing or putting hands together), unique communication patterns and rules (e.g., the use of indirect expressions and the need to read between the lines), and respect and value in certain constructs (e.g., seniority and expertise).

In terms of language, the same word in two different languages may not have the same meaning. For example, the meaning of *leisure* in Japanese refers to organized leisure services such as amusement parks, which is different from the original meaning in English (Iwasaki, Nishino, Onda, & Bowling, 2007). This is because there is no such word to describe *leisure* in traditional Japanese and the word was imported from English in the modern era.

Communication patterns may be strongly influenced by culture. For example, *enryo-sasshi* is a Japanese cultural communication behavior that leads to a modest expression of one's self, and in some cases, vagueness that the information receivers are expected to interpret through sensitive guesswork (Kitano, 1993). Context of the conversation and nonverbal cues are highly important in order to understand the speaker.

Respect and value of seniority and expertise take a form of social hierarchy in Japan and other areas of Asia. In the hierarchy, opposition to the person in the higher position is regarded as a taboo. In a recreational therapy context, the therapist, who has expertise, takes a higher position than the client in the hierarchy. Even if the Japanese client disagrees with what the therapist says, the client may express agreement because opposition to the person in a higher position is not appropriate in their own culture.

As we have discussed in this section, culture takes different forms and plays an important role in the way that assessment is conducted with our clients. This includes the way culture may make communication difficult. There is a risk of misunderstanding between a therapist and a client that might lead to errors in interpreting the assessment results. In addition, the chance of working with clients from diverse cultural backgrounds is increasing due to world demographic changes. Within a global context, migration and cultural changes continue to grow, creating an ever-changing society that requires recreational therapists to be accepting and reflective of diverse communities. It is important to note that many of the concepts discussed in this chapter can also be applied to members of the LGBTQ+ communities due to the existence of different cultures within the larger community. Thus, recreational therapists need to be aware of culture and its influence in assessment. Within this chapter, we provide discussion on the importance of cultural awareness in recreational therapy assessment and provide the reader tangible tools necessary for incorporating culturally sensitive assessment into their practice.

Why an Awareness of Culture Matters

There is an urgent need for us, as practitioners, to prepare for increasingly diverse demographic populations. Clients with diverse cultural backgrounds may not experience positive medical treatment if therapists lack awareness of the clients' cultural needs. From a recreational therapy context, Dieser (2002) wrote of his professional practice experience when the clients he was working with terminated the treatment prematurely because therapists ignored the clients' culture: "[T]he reason why minority-group individuals underutilize and prematurely terminate counseling/therapy lies in the biased nature of the services themselves (i.e., white middle class)" (Dieser, 2002, p. 93). More recently, Dieser (2014) emphasized that recreational therapy textbooks do not cover cross-cultural competence at an adequate level, which may be one of the underlying factors as to why providers fail to address the needs of clients with different cultural backgrounds.

The increase in diversified populations is a result of migration. *Migration* refers to the movement of people from one area to another, such as from Mexico to the United States. Because of this migration, the number of clients from diverse backgrounds receiving recreational therapy service is increasing (Genoe, Hopper, & Singleton, 2017). In addition to migration from one country to another, migration within countries is significant. For instance, migration to areas such as the Midwestern United States, which had been relatively less diverse than other areas in the United States, has been increasing (Fennelly, 2012; Migration Policy Institute, 2017), causing the clientele of health care services to become more culturally diverse. For example, in the Midwest, the Latinx and Asian populations are growing at a rate 12 to 14 times faster than the Caucasian population (Fennelly, 2012).

Given the increase in migration both from outside and inside countries, issues related to culture continue growing in relevance for recreational therapists. This next section discusses at length some of the issues related to culture and recreation therapy practice.

Issues Related to Culture

When a recreational therapist works with a client from a different culture than their own, the therapist might be puzzled with the client's behavior. How do you understand the client? It is helpful for therapists to understand several important concepts that might be associated with client behaviors. In this section, we will discuss these foundational concepts.

Social Dominance

Typically, culture is developed within a group, and the groups constantly interact with each other in a society. In this social process, some groups develop increased power in comparison to other groups, resulting in the formation of a group-based hierarchy and power imbalances in the society. The groups with higher power maintain their power and hierarchy, and groups with lower power attempt to attenuate this inequality. This is a premise of social dominance theory (Sidanius & Pratto, 2012), and it provides helpful insights in order to understand issues related to culture. After the colonial era and two world wars, European and North American groups took higher positions in the hierarchy of many societies. One way to maintain their positions and power was by legitimatizing their culture. The effort was to have people believe that Euro-American culture, including food, lifestyle, and architecture, was superior to other cultures. This was accompanied by a devaluing of the other cultures as primitive or inferior. As a result, people with a different cultural background were marginalized.

In the field of recreational therapy, the majority of recreational therapists are non-Hispanic whites (Stone, 2003). In addition, the recreational therapy curriculum was developed and taught by individuals who were white and from the middle class (Dieser, 2002; 2014). This represents a form of social dominance, legitimatizing the ideology of a white middle class. As discussed by Holland (2014), the field needs diversity in practitioners as well as educators.

Ethnocentrism

Because the field of recreational therapy was developed based on Eurocentric ideology (Dieser, 2002), there are unwritten assumptions in the discipline. One assumption is the belief that our thoughts and beliefs are superior (i.e., Euro-American ideals) and are universally important regardless of culture. This is an example of *ethnocentrism*, which is defined as "the cultural or ethnic bias—whether conscious or unconscious—in which an individual views the world from the perspective of his or her own group, establishing the in-group as archetypal and rating all other groups with reference to this ideal" (Baylor, 2012, p. 1).

Dieser (2002) explained how ethnocentrism can take form in a recreational therapy context through his personal experience working with clients of African American descent in a behavioral health setting. When Dieser conducted an assessment, he determined that the client's interpersonal dependency and lack of self-awareness were problematic based on his Caucasian value system. Dieser (2002) found that African American culture, however, regards interpersonal dependency as desirable. Dieser unconsciously made a biased judgment and problematized what is actually not problematic in the client's own culture. The story demonstrates that we often do not realize our ethnocentrism when we provide culturally inappropriate treatment. Therefore, therapists should critically evaluate whether their recommendations are culturally appropriate for the client.

Cultural Norms: Individualism and Collectivism

When we start paying attention to culture, what might stand out is the cultural tendency to frame lived experiences. For example, Caucasians are often comfortable discussing personal matters, whereas individuals from East Asian countries may not be comfortable asking questions or disagreeing with opinions. In general, we see considerable differences between Westerners—which typically refer to people in North America and Europe—and people from other cultures (Laungani, 2007). The majority of Western cultures possess individualistic orientations, which focuses more on an individual than on a group.

East Asians—typically referring to people in China, Korea, and Japan—have opposite tendencies. East Asian cultures possess col-lectivistic orientations, focusing on the group rather than on an individual. They value group harmony and tend to hold back their own opinions in order to maintain the harmony. Another important difference between individualism and collectivism is the value of independence. Typically, people with individualistic culture value independence, making dependency an undesirable condition in their worldview. In contrast, people with collectivistic culture believe that some degree of dependency is normal or even desirable in order to maintain their group's harmony.

Cultural Assimilation and Ethnic Identity

When an individual immigrates into a country with a different culture, the individual may learn the culture and alter their behaviors. Caldarola, Shimpo, and Ujimoto (2007) studied Japanese Canadians and found that some family members began using English as their primary language. In addition, they adopted Canadian religious architecture and Christianity practices, demonstrating Buddhism-Christianity fusion. However, some Japanese traditions such as food and festivals were widely maintained even within the families who adopted English as their primary language at home.

Acquiring specific cultural attributes of the immigrated country is called *cultural assimilation*. Some, such as the acquisition of the host country's language, could be acquired in a relatively short period of time, but other behaviors, such as educational orientations, what to eat, and ways of thinking, may take a longer time to acquire. There are a variety of degrees of cultural assimilation; thus first-generation immigrants may acquire fewer cultural behaviors than the second and third generations. Understanding cultural background would assist practitioners in helping their clients identify what leisure pursuits may be the most meaningfully engaging. Of particular importance is the connection between cultural connectedness and meaning-making (Iwasaki, Messina, & Hopper, 2018). For example, connecting a client with a cultural community group that regularly facilitates culturally relevant programming would be a beginning point for bridging cultural connectedness and meaning. This participation may evolve into regular engagement in meaningful, cultural leisure.

Ethnic identity is another concern for therapists working with immigrants or individuals from diverse cultural backgrounds. *Ethnic identity* refers to being a member of a specific ethnic group as well as having the qualities of the ethnic group (Masuda, Matsumoto, & Meredith, 1970). Ethnic identity is an important indicator of cultural assimilation, which indicates how much cultural attributes may be maintained within the individual. Among second- and later-generation immigrants, ethnic identity may be diminished because of limited contact with the culture. First-generation immigrants might have stronger ties and interactions with people with the same culture, therefore they have more opportunities to maintain their culture and ethnic identity. However, the second- and later-generation residents may have proportionally fewer opportunities to interact with people from their country of origin (Caldarola, Shimpo, & Ujimoto, 2007). Caldarola and colleagues reported that third-generation Japanese Canadians received assistance such as getting to know their grandparents so that they can maintain their ethnic identity. Previous studies of ethnic identity among Japanese Americans found that the second generation has lower ethnic identity than the first generation, and the third generation has lower ethnic identity than the second (Marsella, Johnson, Johnson, & Brennan, 1998; Masuda, Matsumoto, & Meredith, 1970). While later-generation residents may have physical characteristics of their ancestors' country of origin, they may not be able to speak the language or participate in any of the cultural activities. As a result, later-generation residents may not maintain the ethnic identity of their ancestors' origin. Recreational therapists should investigate the person's ethnic identity instead of making a judgment based on the person's appearance.

Other Factors That Complicate Client Experience of Culture: An Intersectionality Perspective

Identifying the cultural background of your clients is important, but there are countless interactions with other sociodemographic variables such as age, gender, and socioeconomic status, and it is unrealistic to know each and every factor that influences what it means to be in a specific culture. For example, being an immigrant and being in poverty is drastically different from being an immigrant but having enough financial means to get necessities taken care of. The concept of intersectionality (Crenshaw, 1991) is helpful to continually remind ourselves about the complexity of the actual client situations. *Intersectionality* is the idea that disadvantages in life are not rooted in a single factor, but rather are the consequences of multiple factors (Hankivsky, 2014). For example, one's cultural background may not be the only reason for mistreatment—the combination of being a woman and lacking financial means can also contribute. Culture is important, but other factors are required to understand the full picture of a person. Intersectionality is especially appropriate when working with members of the LGBTQ+ communities because multiple factors, like being gay and African American, can contribute to greater mistreatment when compared to identifying with only one of the aforementioned cultures. The potential mistreatment due to race can be compounded by the mistreatment that affects sexual orientation. Awareness of the impact that these differing combinations of culture(s) can have enables a recreational therapist to increase the efficacy and appropriateness of their assessment and treatment.

The world we live in reflects the idea of intersectionality, and it is why the World Health Organization's (WHO) *International Classification of Functioning, Disability and Health* (ICF) (see chapter 3) framework provides an understanding of individual differences among people who share the same culture. Careful study of personal factors give practitioners a guide to understand who the client is, and this information is a key ingredient to create a culturally safe place, where clients feel that their culture is respected.

TR Assessment (Instruments and Process) and Culture

The lack of cultural understanding is a significant factor that undermines valid assessment of our clients. How your client responds to your probes during the interview is significantly influenced by the person's cultural background. When your client is asked an assessment question during the interview, the following things occur: a) The client cognitively processes the words to comprehend what it means; and b) the client outputs the answer to the question. This comprehension and output are done through their cultural filter. The main concerns are whether the client understands the questions asked and whether the therapist understands the client's expressed concerns.

Client's Understanding of the Assessment Questions

One source of cultural bias in assessment is the language. Because some terms used in assessment (such as *leisure*) may have a different meaning across cultures, misunderstanding between the client and the therapist may occur. For example, "leisure" in Japanese refers to commercial leisure (Iwasaki et al., 2007). Therefore, Japanese people may not associate the word *leisure* with commonly practiced leisure activities among Japanese such as walking in a park (*Sanpo*), having a tea with friends (*Ocha*), and attending a community festival (*Matsuri*). As a result, a Japanese client may misunderstand the question and provide an inaccurate answer. One potential approach is to use the client's own language that reflects the meaning of the word, instead of direct translation of the words. By using client's own cultural terminology, therapists can not only deliver

the nuance of the word but also show respect to the client (Iwasaki et al., 2007). If the person was asked with the Japanese terms (i.e., *sanpo*, *ocha*, and *matsuri*), the person could understand that those activities are for fun. In addition, they may be more engaged because they felt respected. This requires some understanding of the client's culture. The work of Holland (2014) explained typical holidays, customs, and recreation of ethnic groups such as African Americans, Chinese Americans, Japanese Americans, Hmong Americans, Mexican Americans, and Puerto Ricans. This could help the recreational therapist gain insight into activities that might interest those individuals.

Because language is a significant source of bias, recreational therapists must examine the instruments they wish to use. Paniagua (2013) introduced a set of questions to assess whether an instrument is culturally sensitive. Relevant questions identified by Paniagua to assist in assessing an instrument are the following:

- Do the concepts the instrument aims to capture exist in the client's culture?
- Do the words used in the items exist in the client's culture?
- Do the words used mean the same thing in the client's culture?
- Do the behaviors of the client (e.g., eye contact, assertiveness) mean the same thing within their culture as in the culture that developed the instrument?

Therapist's Understanding of the Client's Expressed Concerns

Recreational therapists need to be aware how culture may influence their interpretation of the client's response to the questions asked. Here, we will discuss concerns that are helpful when using interviews, observation, and standardized assessment.

Interviews

What a client says should be carefully interpreted with cultural context, because people in some cultures may use a word with a different meaning than the mainstream culture. For example, *yes* usually means approval of an opinion or suggestion in North American usage; however, Japanese speakers use *yes* to mean "I understand," without an implication of approval. This might result in misunderstanding the client's treatment decision by not ascertaining their true feelings.

Another potential pitfall is language proficiency of the client—clients may not be able to express their ideas because they do not know the right words in English, even though they know them in their mother language (Holland, 2014). Therapists need to be sensitive when a client has a difficult time expressing themselves. The use of alternative communication such as a picture board or interpreter can be helpful so that clients can answer the assessment questions to the best of their ability.

Observations

Therapists should be aware that behavioral cues may have different meanings in different cultures. Dieser (2002) shared his experience of misunderstanding behavioral cues such as lack of eye contact within African American culture, which caused inaccurate assessment results (i.e., problematized culturally acceptable behaviors) as well as distrust because the client was forced to work on a culturally inappropriate goal. Some issues can be avoided with basic understanding of the meaning of behavioral cues in certain cultures. If the therapist knows that avoiding eye contact is appropriate within the client's culture, they will know that increasing eye contact is an inappropriate goal for that client.

Standardized Assessment

When interpreting results from standardized assessments, it's helpful to understand the client's cultural norms. For example, people in collectivistic countries such as China, Korea, and Japan are known to have a lower norm score in self-esteem than people in individualistic countries (Kang, Shaver, Sue, Min, & Jing, 2003; Schmitt & Allik, 2005) because people in these cultures usually present themselves modestly in order to maintain the group harmony. Thus, even if a collectivistic individual had a low score in self-esteem, they may be as proud of themselves as an individualistic individual who scored higher. Knowing the norm scores specific to each cultural group will help us avoid problematizing culturally acceptable levels of some measures. In addition, triangulation through interview probing can be helpful as well. Whether or not the client agrees that there is a problem can often be clarified by asking them directly. Sometimes you may find that a low score on a standardized scale does not comprise a problem in their culture.

Applying ICF Framework Into Practice

The ICF provides a helpful perspective for successfully assessing clients with diverse cultural backgrounds. The most relevant part of the ICF is contextual factors, including personal factors. The client's race (defined as biological or genetic) and ethnicity (defined as cultural or social), which are relevant to personal factors, should be noted at the beginning of the process. However, identifying the client's race and ethnicity is not enough. The person's worldview—more specifically, individualism versus collectivism, the extent of cultural assimilation, what pursuits may be associated with the person's meaningful leisure engagement, and personal traits not related to culture—is needed to obtain a full picture of the person.

One approach is to use the Context-Phase-Stage-Style (CPSS) model that was modified for recreational therapy use by Dieser (2014). CPSS can be a helpful guide to assist the recreational therapist during assessment to systematically cover the important areas: Where is the client located on the individualism/collectivism continuum (context); how does the client see themselves in psychosocial phases of cultural assimilation (phase); in what leisure activities does the client meaningfully engage (stage); and what preferences or personality traits influence the client's leisure behavior (style)?

ICF's personal factors are important to make sure the therapist understands the complex social context affected by factors such as age, gender, and socioeconomic status. This perspective particularly addresses intersectionality theory.

Cultural Competence and Cultural Safety

The concept of cultural competence was introduced in order to properly treat health care consumers who are increasingly diverse. Cultural competence is defined as the ability to provide care to clients with diverse values, beliefs, and behaviors, including tailoring delivery to meet patients' social, cultural, and linguistic needs (Betancourt, Green, Carrillo, & Ananeh-Firempong, 2003). Cultural competence is relevant to not only individual therapists but also organizations where the therapists work. In this chapter, we focus primarily on the individual level, but therapists and educators should notice the importance of organizational-level cultural competence. Adopting cultural competence improves trust and satisfaction (Bhui, Warfa, Edonya, McKenzie, & Bhugra, 2007; Paez, Allen, Beach, Carson, & Cooper, 2009) and reduces health disparities (Betancourt, Green, Carrillo, & Park, 2005). For further study, we recommend reviewing cultural competence of the Substance Abuse and Mental Health Services Administration (SAMHSA) (2014). The resource includes a cultural competence self-assessment for professionals, which examines professional cultural awareness, including knowledge and attitudes toward individuals who have diverse backgrounds and the skills to accommodate them. This resource also includes the multicultural intake checklist, which may be a useful guide during an intake interview.

How does an individual gain cultural competence? Purnell (2012) modeled the key milestones of how an individual nurtures his or her cultural competence. These milestones include cultural awareness, cultural sensitivity, and cultural competence. In the first stage, the person needs to be aware of the existence of different cultures and recognize the importance to treat them in a respectful manner. In the second stage, gaining basic understanding of cultures, an individual becomes more careful with things they say and do to others from different cultures. At the last stage, an individual can serve their clients with appropriate care given the clients' cultural background.

Cultural competence is important, but there are some critical limitations, too. First, it is impossible for us to truly understand each and every culture—especially because culture is not concrete but somewhat fluid, even in ourselves. Second, the cultural competence approach tends to be "one size fits all," ignoring variations among the same ethnic background, which promotes stereotypes and results in disempowerment of health care recipients instead.

Some scholars have proposed that medical professionals should instead create *cultural safety* in their practice. Cultural safety is an approach to create a safe place for all health care recipients and involves: a) health care providers' awareness of their own culture; b) health care provider's open mindedness; and c) not blaming victims (Crampton, Dowell, Parkin, & Thompson, 2003). The therapist gives their client an opportunity to tell what is important to them, rather than the therapist assuming what is important to the client. It is true that openness and flexibility are not enough by themselves; however, a cultural safety approach certainly addresses issues that cultural competence cannot solve. By "recognizing the social, historical, political and economic circumstances that create power differences and inequalities in health and the clinical encounter" (Kirmayer, 2012, p. 158), cultural safety can provide truly empowering health care. It is important to note that a combination of intersectionality and the ICF approach can successfully lead to a practice of cultural safety because intersectionality theory (Crenshaw, 1991) helps us understand the many demographic variables of an individual (age, gender, socioeconomic status) instead of stereotyping each and every culture. For example, a therapist who uses the ICF approach will investigate sociodemographic variables, and intersectionality theory makes us ask questions about how different combinations of sociodemographic variables might lead to different experiences.

We recommend practicing cultural safety while developing cultural competence. Cultural safety is very important in theory, but the implications and training are vague and still in development. On the other hand, understanding basic knowledge about different cultures is critically important for identifying areas that require care. Recreational therapy students, practitioners, and educators should recognize and be familiar with both cultural competence and cultural safety.

CASE STUDY

A Snapshot of Serving Clients From Diverse Cultural Backgrounds in a Physical Medicine Setting

Written by Marc Zaremski, MS, CTRS: Clemson University

John is a 56-year-old male from Manila, Philippines. The primary language he speaks at home is Tagalog but he is also fluent in English. John moved from Manila to Florida when he was 13 years old with his parents. John has remained in Florida and he currently lives with his wife and youngest daughter. John's wife speaks Tagalog and some English and his daughter is bilingual. John was working on his roof when he experienced a dizzy spell and fell backward off of the ladder, approximately 15 feet, landing on his driveway. John did not lose consciousness and an ambulance was called immediately once he expressed to his wife that he could not move his legs. John sustained fractures in several thoracic vertebrae from T8 to T12. At the T10 level, he sustained a complete spinal cord injury, resulting in paralysis below the T10 level. The ambulance took him to the local trauma center, where he underwent several procedures to stabilize the spinal cord and relieve pressure at the injury site. After John was deemed medically stable, he was transferred to ABC Rehabilitation to receive inpatient rehabilitation approximately seven days postoperative.

At ABC Rehabilitation, John's therapy and medical teams consist of only English-speaking therapists who are all non-Hispanic Caucasian. The facility offers a translation service, when available, which is a live video feed of a translator that can assist during therapy sessions, doctor's visits, and any other time a patient might need information translated to or from a provider. John initially feels comfortable but some aspects of the hospital begin to conflict with his culture. The constant cold temperature throughout the hospital is concerning to him because he believes warmth promotes good health. John's more traditional relatives have expressed concern over food, the treatment plan, and the temperature of the facility as well. A member of John's family is a *babaylan*, which is a form of healer that uses prayers, herbs, and massage or tissue manipulation as a healing method. John asked his physician and physical therapist if this family member could perform their healing rituals on him. They deemed it unwise because the family member is not a medical professional and John has many precautions. John was disappointed but eventually convinced the medical team to allow this healer to work with him. They agreed, as long as John informed the *babaylan* of his medical precautions to avoid further injury. The healer is not fluent in English and John had difficulties translating some of the medical terminology. The therapy team used the translation service to confirm that the healer and John understand the restrictions of the treatment. John and the healer articulated that they understood the precautions and John was able to participate in this healing session. John enjoyed the healing session and it put his more traditional family members at ease.

Throughout John's stay he experienced some frustrations and setbacks. Some frustrations were because of how his life had changed due to his injury and some were because of language barriers and a lack of specific cultural knowledge from health care providers. With the flexibility and extra effort of his health care professional, John overcame some of these issues to progress into being independent in his wheelchair and was deemed eligible to return home safely.

> continued

CASE STUDY   > continued

It is unrealistic to expect every health care provider to be knowledgeable on the cultural traditions and preferences of every client or patient. But it is important to utilize available resources to gain some insight into what our patients and clients prefer and to find compromise between those beliefs and the best possible medical care.

Applying ICF and Purnell's Stages of Cultural Competence

Based on Purnell's (2012) cultural competence milestones, the level of cultural competence of the physicians and physical therapist does not appear to reach to the cultural sensitivity stage, as evidenced by careless rejections of the healing rituals. They might have noticed that John's background is Filipino; however, they were not aware of how important it was to John and his family members for John to receive healing rituals. In order for physicians and physical therapists to reach a higher stage of cultural competence, the ICF framework is helpful. Personal factors of ICF allow them to look at the person's worldview and value system, beyond race and ethnicity. By understanding the client's values, professionals are more likely to seek ways to achieve things that are important to the person.

Implications for Recreational Therapy Practice

Working with patients or clients from different cultural backgrounds can provide some difficulties for professionals. But many of these difficulties can be resolved or mitigated with extra effort and preparation. Taking the time to look at the resources of your facility and how to access them is a great starting point for establishing a protocol for future clients. If there is admission data or another professional at the facility that may have seen this client first, talking to them can be useful for knowing what resources you may need to acquire. For example, if a patient is admitted who only speaks Spanish, that fact should appear in admission data or a member of the treatment team may inform you prior to you seeing them. This will enable you to schedule that patient when a translator, translation device, or family member that can translate is available. Scheduling appropriately, however, is not a static solution, so a backup plan should be established in case those resources are unavailable. Online translators can be useful for getting some basic translations to assist in your sessions. When all resources are unavailable, a list of key translated words to assist in administering the intervention for that day or for their length of stay may be required. It is difficult to coordinate translation services throughout an entire length of a patient's stay, so having these backup words can be vital for continuing quality service delivery.

Information on those you serve is vital for providing quality care. But it is also important to remember that something you may have found to be true for one patient may not be true for another, even if they have similar backgrounds. The Internet can be useful for finding information on cultures and their traditions, but it is safer to not to make assumptions. The best source of information on your client's beliefs, traditions, and background is typically from the client or their close family members and friends.

Being an active listener allows you to hear concerns that your client may have. This opens up an opportunity for recreational therapists to mitigate those concerns that could be making the client feel uncomfortable. For example, at some facilities, the recreational therapist may have the opportunity to do cooking or kitchen interventions. On occasion, a patient will have religious or cultural dietary restrictions and the food service department may not be meeting these needs. Members of the recreation department should perform functional cooking tasks with patients that meet their religious or cultural needs. This can make the patient or client feel more comfortable during their stay and assist other medical providers in meeting their goals for the client or patient.

When working with patients or clients from diverse cultural backgrounds, the best strategy for working with them can be broken down into four parts:

1. Take extra time to gather and access resources.
2. Utilize all available data and information.
3. Listen to the patient and their caregiver(s) and family members.
4. Work to minimize any of the client's concerns.

To help yourself, it can be beneficial to write down or keep stock of the resources and strategies that were most effective for a given scenario. Using these strategies, a solid foundation can be made to assist recreational therapists in better serving populations from diverse cultural backgrounds.

Questions for Consideration

1. What strategies did the treatment team use in order to understand John?
2. Based on the descriptions of John, to what extent was John culturally assimilated?
3. Viewing this case study through an intersectionality lens, what sociodemographic variables might be helpful to understand John?
4. If you were a member of John's therapy team, what would you do to implement cultural safety?
5. In what way can practitioners move up the stages of cultural competence? How are ICF's personal factors helpful in the process?

Summary

This chapter provided an overview of culture and how recreational therapists might conduct more accurate and successful assessments through cultural sensitivity. The rate of clients who have diverse cultural backgrounds in recreational therapy settings will continue to increase as a result of world demographic changes. Culture does influence communication patterns, and misunderstanding can be avoided with an understanding of the culture of our clientele. When working with clients who have diverse cultural backgrounds, therapists should work to be more aware of unconscious ethnocentrism. Other issues that are important to understand are the differences between individualism and collectivism, cultural assimilation, and intersectionality theory.

When conducting assessments, there might be problems with how well the client understands the assessment questions and how the therapist interprets the answer. Careful examination of the assessment questions is essential, and the use of the clients' terms may improve communication. In addition, research on the cultural norms of the client can avoid problematizing an appropriate behavior based on the client's culture. ICF's personal factors are most relevant to cultural issues and must be thoroughly examined in order to address intersectionality. Furthermore, the CPSS model (Dieser, 2014) might be helpful to ensure recreational therapists cover all the important areas regarding culture. In conclusion, this chapter discussed issues of cultural competence and cultural safety in the assessment process to ensure successful accommodation of clients from diverse cultural backgrounds.

REFLECTION QUESTIONS

1. What is the definition of culture? What are some examples of culture? Why is an awareness of culture important for recreational therapists?
2. Have you ever experienced exclusion based on your values, beliefs, or behavior? What could be done to create a culturally safe place for you?

3. Have you seen any examples of ethnocentrism? Did the person act like that intentionally?

4. Think about your thoughts, feelings, and behaviors in the past few weeks. To what extent do you see individualistic and collectivistic tendencies?

5. Think back to a time when your conversation partner did not understand your question. Why did it happen? How did you fix the problem so that your conversation partner could understand?

6. Define cultural competence and cultural safety. What are the differences between them? Which approach would you take when you work with your clients?

REFERENCES

Baylor, E. (2012). Ethnocentrism. *Oxford Bibliographies.* Retrieved from www.oxfordbibliographies.com/view/document/obo-9780199766567/obo-9780199766567-0045.xml

Betancourt, J.R., Green, A.R., Carrillo, J.E., & Ananeh-Firempong, O. (2003). Defining cultural competence: A practical framework for addressing racial/ethnic disparities in health and health care. *Public Health Reports, 118,* 293-302.

Betancourt, J.R., Green, A.R., Carrillo, J.E., & Park, E.R. (2005). Cultural competence and health care disparities: Key perspectives and trends. *Health Affairs, 24*(2), 499-505.

Bhui, K., Warfa, N., Edonya, P., McKenzie, K., & Bhugra, D. (2007). Cultural competence in mental health care: A review of model evaluations. *BMC Health Services Research, 7*(1), 15.

Caldarola, C., Shimpo, M., & Ujimoto, V. (2007). *Sakura in the land of the maple leaf: Japanese cultural traditions in Canada.* Gatineau, QC: Canadian Museum of Civilization Corporation.

Crampton, P., Dowell, A., Parkin, C., & Thompson, C. (2003). Combating effects of racism through a cultural immersion medical education program. *Academic Medicine, 78*(6), 595-598.

Crenshaw, K. (1991). Mapping the margins: Intersectionality, identity politics, and violence against women of color. *Stanford Law Review, 43*(6), 1241-1299.

Dieser, R.B. (2002). A personal narrative of a cross-cultural experience in therapeutic recreation: Unmasking the masked. *Therapeutic Recreation Journal, 36*(1), 84-96.

Dieser, R.B. (2014). Cross-cultural assessment in therapeutic recreation. *Therapeutic Recreation Journal, 48*(1), 1-14.

Fennelly, K. (2012). *Immigration in the Midwest.* Scholars Strategy Network Basic Facts. Retrieved from www.scholarsstrategynetwork.org/brief/immigration-midwest

Genoe, R., Hopper, T., & Singleton, J.F. (2017). World demographics and their implications for therapeutic recreation. In N.J. Stumbo, B.D. Wolfe, & S. Pegg (Eds.), *Professional issues in therapeutic recreation: On competence and outcomes* (3rd ed., pp. 57-66). Urbana-Champaign, IL: Sagamore Publishing.

Griswold, W. (2013). *Cultures and societies in the changing world.* Los Angeles, CA: Sage Publications.

Hankivsky, O. (2014). *Intersectionality 101.* Burnaby, BC: The Institute for Intersectionality Research & Policy, Simon Fraser University. Retrieved from www.sfu.ca/iirp/documents/resources/101_Final.pdf

Holland, J.W. (2014). *Cultural competence in recreational therapy.* Enumclaw, WA: Idyll Arbor.

Iwasaki, Y., Messina, E., & Hopper, T. (2018). The role of leisure in meaning-making and engagement with life. *Journal of Positive Psychology, 1,* 29-35.

Iwasaki, Y., Nishino, H., Onda, T., & Bowling, C. (2007). Leisure research in a global world: Time to reverse the western domination in leisure research? *Leisure Sciences, 29*(1), 113-117.

Kang, S.M., Shaver, P.R., Sue, S., Min, K.H., & Jing, H. (2003). Culture-specific patterns in the prediction of life satisfaction: Roles of emotion, relationship quality, and self-esteem. *Personality and Social Psychology Bulletin, 29*(12), 1596-1608.

Kirmayer, L.J. (2012). Rethinking cultural competence. *Transcultural Psychiatry, 49*(2), 149-164.

Kitano, H.L. (1993). Japanese American values and communication patterns. In W.B. Gudykunst (Ed.), *Communication in Japan and the United States* (pp. 122-148). Albany, NY: SUNY Press.

Laungani, P. (2007). *Understanding cross-cultural psychology.* London, UK: Sage Publication.

Marsella, A.J., Johnson, F.A., Johnson, C.L., & Brennan, J. (1998). Ethnic identity in second (Nisei), third (Sansei), and fourth (Yonsei) generation Japanese Americans in

Hawaii. *Asian American and Pacific Islander Journal of Health, 6*(1), 46-52.

Masuda, M., Matsumoto, G.H., & Meredith, G.M. (1970). Ethnic identity in three generations of Japanese Americans. *The Journal of Social Psychology, 81*(2), 199-207.

Migration Policy Institute. (2017). U.S. immigrant population and share over time, 1850–present. Retrieved from www.migrationpolicy.org/programs/data-hub/charts/immigrant-population-over-time

Paez, K.A., Allen, J.K., Beach, M.C., Carson, K.A., & Cooper, L.A. (2009). Physician cultural competence and patient ratings of the patient-physician relationship. *Journal of General Internal Medicine, 24*(4), 495-498.

Paniagua, F.A. (2013). *Assessing and treating culturally diverse clients: A practical guide* (4th ed.). Thousand Oaks, CA: Sage.

Purnell, L.D. (2012). *Transcultural health care: A culturally competent approach.* Philadelphia, PA: FA Davis.

Schmitt, D.P., & Allik, J. (2005). Simultaneous administration of Rosenberg self-esteem scale in 53 nations: Exploring the universal and cultural-specific features of global self-esteem. *Journal of Personality and Social Psychology, 89*(4), 623-642.

Sidanius, J., & Pratto, F. (2012). Social dominance theory. In P.M. Van Lange, A.W. Kruglanski, & E.T. Higgins (Eds.), *Handbook of theories of social psychology, volume 1* (pp. 418-438). Thousand Oaks, CA: Sage Publications.

Stone, C.F. (2003). Exploring cultural competencies of certified therapeutic recreation specialists: Implications for education and training. *Therapeutic Recreation Journal, 37*(2), 156-174.

Substance Abuse and Mental Health Services Administration (SAMHSA). (2014). *Improving cultural competence: A treatment improvement protocol.* (HHS Publication No. (SMA) 14-4849). Rockville, MD: Author.

ADDITIONAL RESOURCES

Aho, J. (2007). Therapeutic recreation in Finland. *Therapeutic Recreation Journal, 41*(2), 141-147.

Commission and Accreditation of Allied Health Education Programs (CAAHEP). (2017). Recreational therapy standards. Retrieved from www.caahep.org/getattachment/About-CAAHEP/Committees-on-Accreditation/Recreational-Therapy/2017-Recreational-Therapy-Standards.pdf.aspx

Geva, E. (2015). *Psychological assessment of culturally and linguistically diverse children and adolescents: A practitioner's guide.* New York: Springer.

Holland, J.W. (2014). *Cultural competence in recreational therapy.* Enumclaw, WA: Idyll Arbor.

National Council for Therapeutic Recreation Certification (NCTRC). (2016). *Certification standards part V: NCTRC national job analysis.* New York, NY: Author.

Nishino, H.J., Chino, H., Yoshioka, N., & Gabriella, J. (2007). Therapeutic recreation in modern Japan: Era of challenge and opportunity. *Therapeutic Recreation Journal, 41*(2), 119-131.

Paniagua, F.A. (2013). *Assessing and treating culturally diverse clients: A practical guide* (4th ed.). Thousand Oaks, CA: Sage.

Pegg, S., & Darcy, S. (2006). Sailing in troubled water: Diversional therapy in Australia. *Therapeutic Recreation Journal, 41*(2), 132-140.

CHAPTER 10

Final Reflections

Thomas K. Skalko, PhD, LRT/CTRS, FDRT

Jerome F. Singleton, PhD, CTRS

This text builds upon the entry to practice knowledge domains for RT professionals and insights from RT practitioners into assessment. King (2014) illustrated the variety of inputs the recreational therapist needs to include in the assessment process and the provision of specific and comprehensive program design. This text is aimed at advancing the competencies of developing recreational therapy practitioners in the assessment process within the context of the World Health Organization's *International Classification for Functioning, Disability and Health* (ICF). The text integrates the ICF and the assessment process.

The integration of the assessment process with the *International Classification for Functioning, Disability and Health* (ICF) offers recreational therapy professionals multiple levels of information to infuse their services with contemporary practice. The ICF serves as a foundational model for understanding the classification of disabling conditions as a means to focus assessment outcomes and treatment objectives.

This text reinforces that the ICF has several purposes. For instance, the ICF can ultimately be used to track and record data to promote effective service delivery. It can also serve as a research tool to measure outcomes, including quality of life and environmental assets and barriers. Social policy is included in the applications of the ICF in the planning of laws, social security considerations, and architectural planning and design. Finally, the ICF can be used in "needs assessment, matching treatments with specific conditions, vocational assessment, rehabilitation and outcome evaluation" (WHO, 2001, p. 5). The ICF provides a common language for describing health and health-related states in order to improve communication among different users across different disciplines. Through the use of the ICF in the assessment process, outcomes will be better identified for interprofessional planning on behalf of the consumer.

Assessment is a process of including information from multiple perspectives to understand the person's abilities (King, 2014;

WHO, 2001). The text frames the Assess, Plan, Implement, and Evaluate (APIE) process in an application approach.

Linking the Comprehensive Recreational Therapy Service Delivery model (figure 10.1) with the ICF (figure 10.2) provides practitioners with the understanding that assessment is a process that requires multiple information inputs to determine the functional capacities of the individual.

The CRTSD model emphasizes the need for recreational therapy practitioners to view their service delivery as an entire process with multiple strategies that parallel and complement the *International Classification for Functioning, Disability and Health* (ICF).

The ICF model (see figure 10.2) offers a way to classify functioning to ensure the individual receives appropriate services to promote engagement in the life of the community.

The application of basic service delivery approaches, such as utilizing valid and reliable assessment practices, focusing on outcomes consistent with the ICF, and emphasizing a complete understanding of the consumer from their own perspective, is addressed. In addition, the application of task analysis to tailor treatment outcomes compatible with the ICF and the dissemination of evidence-based strategies are all included in the CRTSD model.

By utilizing the ICF and the CRTSD models, the recreational therapist is better prepared

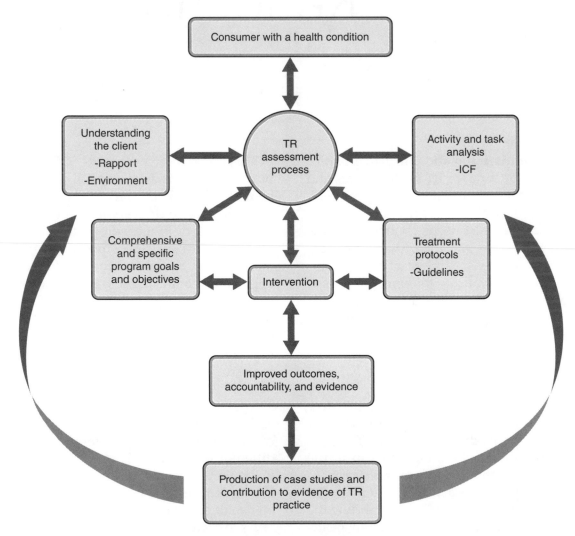

FIGURE 10.1   Model for Comprehensive Recreational Therapy Service Delivery.
King, Singleton, and Skalko, 2018

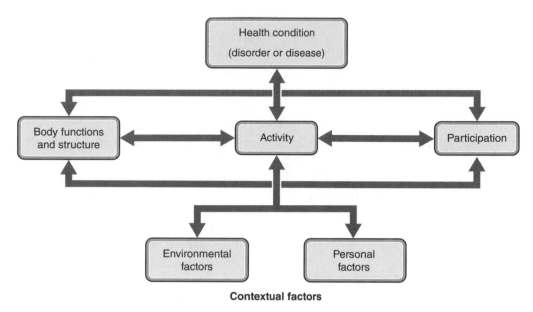

FIGURE 10.2   ICF model.

Reprinted by permission from *International Classification of Functioning, Disability and Health*, pg. 17, copyright 2001 (Geneva, World Health Organization).

to address the complexities of the consumer assessment process. This understanding must include factors such as the consumer's participation in the community (learning and applying knowledge, mobility, major life areas), their physical needs (body functions and structure), and the contextual factors (environmental and personal) of the person within his or her society (WHO, 2001, p. 18). Each of the authors used the ICF model to provide insights into the multiple methods required to understand the person in relation to the ICF domains of Body Structure, Body Function, Activities and Participation, and the Environment, with the ultimate goal of active engagement in the life of the community—the ultimate goal of all rehabilitation disciplines.

Chapters 5 through 9 aid the reader in developing the knowledge and skills to apply contemporary assessment approaches by diagnostic-related groups or service areas. They also facilitate the inclusion of the ICF into the recreational therapy assessment processes.

By including the *International Classification of Functioning, Disability and Health* (ICF) in the assessment process, the recreational therapist is better prepared to interface with other allied health professionals and to focus on treatment outcomes consistent with assessment results and codes of the ICF. In addition, the utilization of the ICF within the assessment process places the individual in social and cultural context that examines the interactions of health and social conditions on a person with a disability through a biopsychosocial model. The ICF also provides the RT professional access to a systematic process of understanding the functional capacity of the person while engaged in an activity. Access to the ICF enables RT professionals to use this information in their assessment. The ICF model focuses on the health condition (disorder or disease), participation in the community (learning and applying knowledge, mobility, major life areas), physical factors (body functions and structure), and contextual factors (environmental, personal) of the person within their lived environment.

The Outcome

We trust you found that each chapter developed your knowledge, skills, and abilities in the assessment process and its connection to the *International Classification for Functioning, Disability and Health*. Students and practitioners will find foundational knowledge on the

ICF, consumer assessment, and the complex nature of assessment when serving the public. Assessment is a multifaceted task regardless of setting, and it is incumbent on the practitioner to attend to the complexities of each individual client assessment.

Each chapter brings to light the underlying concepts of assessment by population and the interrelatedness of the assessment process and the ICF. Case studies, discussion questions, and learning activities were included throughout in order to facilitate the readers' competencies in recreational therapy assessment.

Future Evolutions by the World Health Organization

The World Health Organization (WHO) is continuing its engagement in refining the *International Classification of Functioning, Disability and Health* (ICF) and has introduced the *International Classification of Health Interventions* (ICHI). The ICHI offers a means to identify health interventions that promote the functional outcomes of the ICF.

As delineated by the WHO, the ICHI is "being developed to provide a common tool for reporting and analyzing health interventions for statistical purposes" (WHO, 2018a, p. 1). To promote application, the ICHI identifies a health intervention as "an act performed for, with or on behalf of a person or population whose purpose is to assess, improve, maintain, promote or modify health, functioning or health conditions" (WHO, 2018a, p. 1). Included in the ICHI are interventions implemented across a broad range of providers, addressing the full spectrum of health care systems (e.g., acute care, primary care, rehabilitation, assistance with functioning, prevention, and public health) (WHO, 2018a).

The ICHI utilizes three axes: "Target (the entity on which the Action is carried out), Action (a deed done by an actor to a target) and Means (the processes and methods by which the Action is carried out)" (WHO, 2018a, p. 1). So, the ICHI is designed to assist in identifying *who* will receive the intervention, *what* the health care provider will do with the recipient

of the intervention, and *how* the intervention will be employed.

Similar to the ICF, the ICHI will provide extension codes "to allow users to describe additional detail about the intervention in addition to the relevant ICHI code" (WHO, 2018a, p. 1). At the current time, the ICHI employs a simple classification for international use and eventual international comparisons. Though currently in development, the ICHI will eventually bring to the forefront evidence-based interventions designed to address the assessed functional performance of the individual and the classifications identified within the ICF.

In addition to the ICHI, the World Health Organization is in the process of updating the *International Classification of Diseases* (ICD) from the ICD-10 to the ICD-11. "The ICD is the foundation for identifying health trends and statistics worldwide, and contains around 55,000 unique codes for injuries, diseases and causes of death. It provides a common language that allows health professionals to share health information across the globe" (WHO, 2018b, p. 1). The ICD is used by many health insurance providers to code health conditions for reimbursement purposes and to ultimately track health conditions and allocate resources accordingly. It is important for recreational therapists to possess some familiarity with the ICF, the ICHI, and the ICD to gain a full understanding of the health coding labyrinth.

Implications for the Therapist

This text was designed to promote the integration of recreational therapy assessment within the context of the *International Classification of Functioning, Disability and Health*. It will be incumbent on the individual practitioner to remain current and to develop the knowledge, skills, and abilities to utilize a comprehensive approach to assessment. This will include the integration of valid and reliable assessment data in order to employ the ICF, the ICHI, and the ICD-11.

Today, even familiarity with the ICF remains a challenge for the profession, much less fully understanding the interrelatedness of the ICD and the ICHI. Continuing professional development is essential if recreational therapists are to remain competent and competitive within the health care workforce. Being able to speak the same language, understand and apply valid and reliable assessment processes, and utilize evidence-based intervention strategies will be the hallmark in the future of health care practice.

This text started with insights from RT professionals on the complexities of the assessment process. It links consumer assessment to the ICF and assists RT professionals to understand the complexities of the assessment process within a global context that will assist in interdisciplinary team communication. The ICI II builds upon the ICF and, in conjunction with the ICD-11, will provide the readers of the text with knowledge to apply this framework to service delivery.

The ultimate challenge is for the recreational therapist to remain current in practice and to strive to expand their knowledge base in the assessment process and in the evolution of the ICF, the ICHI, and the ICD-11. You can be assured that professional colleagues in the other disciplines are already integrating these concepts into their practices.

REFERENCES

King, A. (2014). *The pick of the litter? Understanding standardized assessment tools and the assessment process with older adults in therapeutic recreation practitioners* (Master's thesis). Dalhousie University, Halifax.

World Health Organization. (2001). *International classification of functioning, disability and health*. Geneva: Author.

World Health Organization. (2018a). International classification of health interventions. Retrieved from www.who.int/classifications/ichi/en/

World Health Organization. (2018b). WHO releases new International Classification of Diseases (ICD-11). Retrieved July 23, 2018, from www.who.int/newsroom/detail/18-06-2018-who-releases-new-international-classification-of-diseases-(icd-11)

MEDICAL CHARTING ABBREVIATIONS LIST

Abbreviation	Meaning	Abbreviation	Meaning
(A)	assist	CHI	closed head injury
ABD	abduction	C/I	complete independence
a.c.	before meals	c/o	complains of
ADA	Americans with Disabilities Act	CRO	community reintegration outing
ADD	adduction	C.T.R.S. or CTRS	certified therapeutic recreation specialist
A & D	alcohol and drug	cu	cubic
ADL	activities of daily living	CVA	cerebrovascular accident
AFO	ankle–foot orthosis	CVC	central venous catheter
AK	above knee		
AMA	against medical advice	(D) or Dep.	dependent
amb.	ambulation	d/c	discontinue
amp.	amputation	D/C	discharge
B & B	bowel and bladder	DD	developmental disability
b/c	because	DJD	degenerative joint disease
bid	twice a day	DME	durable medical equipment
Bil.	bilateral	DNR	do not resuscitate
BM	bowel movement	DOB	date of birth
BP	blood pressure	DOI	date of injury
C	cervical	DS	discharge summary
c̄	with	DT	delirium tremens
cath	catheterize	DVT	deep vein thrombosis
cc	cubic centimeter (=1 ml)	Dx	diagnosis
C/D	complete dependence	ELOS	estimated length of stay
CD	chemical dependency	ETOH	alcohol
CG	contact guard	EVAL	evaluation
C.H.D.	coronary heart disease	FIM	functional independence measure
CHF	congestive heart failure	F/U	follow-up

(continued)

MEDICAL CHARTING ABBREVIATIONS LIST *(continued)*

Abbreviation	Meaning	Abbreviation	Meaning
func.	functional	m.	meter
Fx or fx	fracture	max.	maximal
GSW	gunshot wound	Max Ⓐ	maximal assistance
h/o	history of	Ⓜ/D	modified dependence
HOH	hard of hearing	MD	muscular dystrophy
H & P	history and physical	mg.	milligram
hr.	hour	Ⓜ/I	modified independence
ht. or ht	height	min.	minimal
Hx. or hx	history	Min Ⓐ	minimal assistance
Ⓘ	independent	ml.	milliliter
IA	initial assessment	mm.	millimeter
ICU	intensive care unit	mod.	moderate
IP	inpatient	Mod Ⓐ	moderate assistance
isol.	isolation	MRI	magnetic resonance imaging
ITP	individual treatment plan	MS	multiple sclerosis
IV	intravenous	N/A	not applicable
kg.	kilogram	NKA	no known allergies
L.	liter	NPO	nothing by mouth
L	lumbar	NSG	nursing
Ⓛ	left	N & V	nausea and vomiting
lat.	lateral	NWB	non-weight bearing (as in crutch walking)
lb.	pound	OD	overdose
LBP	low back pain	OOB	out of bed
LD	learning disability	OP	outpatient
LDB	Leisure Diagnostic Battery	O.T. or OT	occupational therapy
LE	lower extremity	oz.	ounce (30 ml.)
L.E.	leisure education	P	pulse
LLB	long leg brace	p̄	after
ⓁLE	left lower extremity	para	paraplegic
LOS	length of stay	PCN	penicillin
LTG	long-term goal	p.o. or po	by mouth
ⓁUE	left upper extremity		

Abbreviation	Meaning	Abbreviation	Meaning
p.r.n. or PRN	as needed	STG	short term goals
PT or P.T.	physical therapy	S.W. or SW	social work
Pt. or pt	patient	T	thoracic
PWB	partial weight bearing	Ⓣ/A	total assistance
q	every	T.B.I. or TBI	traumatic brain injury
qd	every day	t'fers or t/f	transfer
qh	every hour	tid or t.i.d.	three times daily
qid	four times a day	T.R. or TR	therapeutic recreation
q.o.d.	every other day	TRS	therapeutic recreation specialist
q.o.p.m.	every other night	TWB	total weight bearing
Ⓡ	right	Tx	treatment
RA	rheumatoid arthritis	UE	upper extremity
rec'd	received	UTI	urinary tract infection
ⓇLE	right lower extremity	vo or VO	verbal order
RN	registered nurse	W/C or w/c	wheelchair
ROM	range of motion	WFL	within functional limits
RT	respiratory therapy	wk	week
Rec. Tx. or R.T. or RT	recreation therapy/recreation therapist	WNL	within normal limits
ⓇUE	right upper extremity	wt. or wt	weight
Rx	prescription	x	times; frequency (x3, 4x)
s̄	without	↑	increase
Ⓢ	supervision or setup	↓	decrease
s/b	stand by	@	at
S. B.	spina bifida	Δ	change
SCI	spinal cord injury	≈	approximately
s.o.	standing order	φ	no
s.o.b. or SOB	shortness of breath	2°	secondary to
S.T.	speech therapy	ψ	psychiatric services

TASK ANALYSIS FOR BUYING A COKE FROM A MACHINE WITH A DOLLAR BILL

Instructions

1. Prompt the individual to "Buy a Coke."
2. Walk the individual through all of the following steps, one at a time.
3. If the individual is able to complete the step independently, indicate with a "+", and observe them as they move to the next step.
4. If the individual is unable to complete the step independently, indicate with a "−", assist the individual with the step, and observe them as they move to the next step.
5. Count the independently completed steps for each session and report as a percentage.

1. Locate Coke machine	+									
2. Take wallet out of pocket	−									
3. Take a one dollar bill out of wallet	−									
4. Place the dollar in the dollar slot	−									
5. Press "Coke"	−									
6. If change falls, remove the change	−									
7. Remove the can of Coke from the machine	−									
8. Open the can of Coke	−									
9. Drink the Coke	+									
10. Deposit can in the recycling bin	−									
Session number	1	2	3	4	5	6	7	8	9	

TASK/DISCREPANCY ANALYSIS FOR RIDING THE LIFECYCLE AT THE FITNESS CENTER

Instructions

1. Walk the individual through each of the steps and assess their ability to complete the steps independently by placing a "+" in the middle column for each step that they can complete without assistance.
2. For each step that they are unable to complete independently, place a "−" in the middle column.
3. For each step that they are unable to complete independently, provide a strategy for overcoming this deficit.
4. Strategies may include teaching the skill, modifying the step, providing physical assistance, etc.

Travel to the fitness center.	−	Family member drives Individual learns to use Uber
Enter the building and hand card to attendant.	−	Repetitive practice with modeling
Enter the locker room.	+	
Remove clothes and hang clothes in locker.	+	
Put on gym clothes and tie shoes.	−	Use task analysis to teach these skills
Close and lock locker.	−	Use task analysis to teach how to open combination lock Switch to a lock with a key
Walk to weight room.	+	
Program LifeCycle for 30 minutes.	−	Use task analysis to teach how to program LifeCycle
Ride LifeCycle for 30 minutes.	−	Employ shaping by starting out with 10 minutes and gradually building to 30 minutes
Dismount LifeCycle and wipe it off.	+	

BRIDGEWAY APARTMENTS LEISURE INTEREST ASSESSMENT

Created by Kelly Lopez and Shelley Holland through the support of the Mississippi Council on Developmental Disabilities

Name: _____   Instructor: _____

Date: _____

For each activity listed below, indicate interest by circling **C** for **C**urrently Participating or **I** for Interested in Participating.

Fitness rating	Activity: Fitness room	Interest	Comments
	Walk on treadmill	C I	
	Run on treadmill	C I	
	Ride exercise bicycle	C I	
	Lift free weights (2-6 lbs)	C I	
	Lift weights on universal machine (arms/legs)	C I	

Fitness rating	Activity: Game room/rec room	Interest	Comments
	Play pool	C I	
	Play air hockey	C I	
	Play Wii video games:	C I	
	Strength training	C I	
	Aerobics	C I	
	Yoga	C I	
	Balance	C I	
	Bowling	C I	
	Tennis	C I	
	Trivia	C I	
	Shuffleboard	C I	
	Baseball	C I	
	Golf	C I	
	Boxing	C I	
	Play Wii dance video games	C I	
	Play Wii Brunswick Pro Bowling	C I	
	Walk to Leslie Samsone walking video	C I	

INDEX

Note: The italicized f and t following page numbers refer to figures and tables, respectively.

Thomas Skalko, PhD, LRT/CTRS, FDRT, is a professor emeritus in the College of Health and Human Performance at East Carolina University. Skalko earned his bachelor's and master's degrees in education from the University of Georgia and his doctorate from the University of Maryland. Thomas' background includes direct services in community mental health, inpatient behavioral health, inpatient pediatrics, and primitive therapeutic camping. Thomas is a past president of the American Therapeutic Recreation Association (ATRA) and of the Commission on Accreditation of Allied Health Education Programs (CAAHEP). Skalko is also a past chair of the Committee on Accreditation of Recreational Therapy Education (CARTE) and of the North Carolina Board of Recreational Therapy Licensure (NCBRTL). Photo courtesy of East Carolina University.

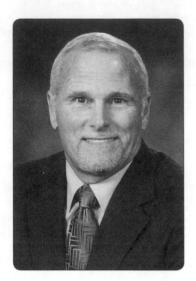

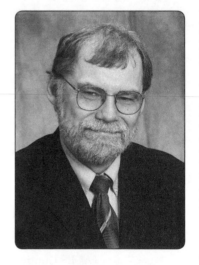

Jerome Singleton, PhD, CTRS, retired in 2018 after 37 years as a professor of recreation and leisure studies in the School of Health and Human Performance at Dalhousie University. He was also cross-appointed to the Schools of Nursing, Sociology and Anthropology, and Business Administration at Dalhousie. He earned his bachelor's degree in recreation from the University of Waterloo, his master's degree in recreation from Pennsylvania State University, and his PhD in leisure studies from the University of Maryland. He also completed the academic requirements for a doctorate certificate in gerontology at the University of Maryland.

Singleton was made a fellow of the World Demographic Association in 2006 and was named Canadian Therapeutic Recreation Association Professional of the Year in 2007. He was recognized by the Recreation and Leisure Studies program at the University of Waterloo as a Distinguished Alumnus in 2008 and is also the founding member of the Leisure and Aging Research Group, which was established in 2008. Singleton received the Dr. Gonzaga da Gama Memorial Award from the Canadian Therapeutic Recreation Association in 2011 and was made a fellow of the Academy of Leisure Science by the Society of Park and Recreation Educators in 2011. Photo courtesy of Jerome Singleton.

CONTRIBUTORS

Frederick Green, PhD, CTRS
Professor
University of Southern Mississippi

Tristan Hopper, PhD, CTRS
Assistant Professor
University of Regina

Christina Jacobs, LMSW
Clinical Therapist

Megan C. Janke, PhD, LRT/CTRS
Associate Professor
East Carolina University

Andrea King, MA, CTRS
Recreation Therapist
Stroke/Neurology Service, Halifax Infirmary

David P. Loy, PhD, LRT/CTRS
Associate Professor
East Carolina University

Bryan P. McCormick, PhD, CTRS
Professor
Temple University

Shinichi Nagata, PhD, CTRS
Assistant Professor
Northwest Missouri State University

Jerome F. Singleton, PhD, CTRS
Professor Emeritus
Dalhousie University

Thomas K. Skalko, PhD, LRT/CTRS, FDRT
Professor Emeritus
East Carolina University

Gretchen Snethen, PhD, CTRS
Associate Professor and Recreational Therapy
Graduate Program Coordinator
Temple University

Marieke Van Puymbroeck, PhD, CTRS, FDRT
Roy Distinguished Professor and Recreational
Therapy Coordinator
Clemson University

Marc Zaremski, MS, CTRS
Clemson University

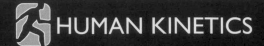
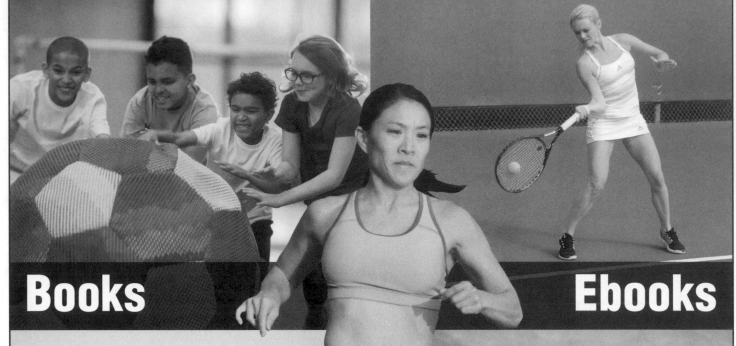
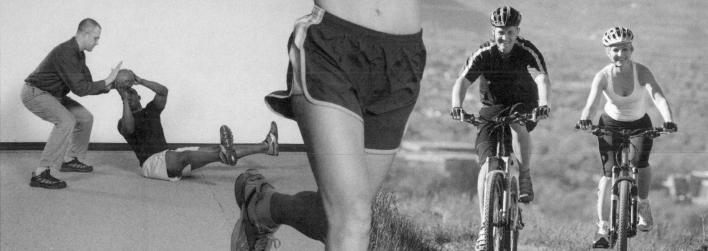